General Editor: C. Vaughan James

MEDICINE

David V. James

MA, MBBS, MRCPsych

TEACHER'S BOOK

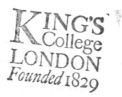

ENGLISH LANGUAGE TEACHING

Prentice Hall

New York   London   Toronto   Sydney   Tokyo   Singapore

First published 1993 by
Prentice Hall Europe
Campus 400, Maylands Avenue
Hemel Hempstead
Hertfordshire, HP2 7EZ
A division of
Simon & Schuster International Group

First published 1989 by Cassell Publishers Limited.

A series design by Passim Ltd, Oxford, and Associates.

British Library Cataloguing in Publication Data

Information available from the publisher on
request.

Medicine Students' Book   0-13-280363-1
Cassettes   0-13-280389-5

3 4 5   97

INTRODUCTION

AIM
The aim of this course is to prepare students in tertiary education to undertake a course in Medicine through the medium of English.

COMPONENTS
The materials consist of this Teacher's Guide, a Students' Book and two cassettes.

LENGTH
The course provides material for approximately 150 lessons, depending on the strength/weakness of the group.

STRUCTURE
The course is divided into 15 units. At the end of Units 5 and 10 there is a Progress Check Test, designed to enable students to check the progress they are making.

STRUCTURE OF A UNIT
The 15 Units are divided into the following eight sections:

A. Understanding a printed text (1)

Each Unit starts with a text of approximately two pages.

Handle the text in two distinct stages:

● Reading for gist
● Reading for detailed understanding

In the first stage, students should concentrate on the general structure of the text from the point of view of its coherence, paying special attention to features such as its title, the notes in the margin, its paragraphing and visuals. They should aim to answer the general questions given at the beginning of the text only, without being distracted by detail — not understanding individual words, for example.

When this has been done, work through the text with the students to ensure detailed understanding. Students should be encouraged to use a dictionary or other reference book when working with the text.

B. Check your understanding

This section consists of a number of questions on the details of the text, and therefore checks detailed understanding.

C. Increase your vocabulary

This section concentrates on the vocabulary details of the text. It consists of a variety of exercises, such as finding synonyms and antonyms, giving explanations of particular terms and so on.

D. Check your grammar

The course assumes that the student will have covered the grammar of English in his/her previous education, but recognises that there may be some elements that require revision. This section therefore provides exercises in some of the key structures of English, and also practice in sentence and paragraph writing. The emphasis is on those features of English that are particularly frequent in 'scientific' writing.

E. Understanding a lecture

This section consists of lecture extracts. Each extract is divided into sections, and there are questions in the Students' Book on each section. There is a variety of questions, such as labelling diagrams, correct/incorrect and so on.

At the end of each lecture, the student is asked to listen to the lecture again and take notes. When this has been done, he/she should write a summary of the lecture, using the notes and the answers to the questions they have already answered.

You should check the notes that students have taken before they write their summaries. If the notes taken are incorrect, go back over the recording again, concentrating on those parts that have been misunderstood.

F. Understanding a printed text (2)

This text continues the topic of the Unit, and should be used to concentrate on detailed understanding.

G. Check your understanding

As in Section A, there is a range of exercises designed to check detailed comprehension of the text.

H. Understanding discourse

This section provides practice in understanding specific directions, instructions (such as books to be read), advice on examinations and so on. Questions are provided in the Student's Book.

Progress check tests

These tests are designed to provide the student with an opportunity to check his/her progress with the course. They consist of the same kind of activities as the Units, namely a Reading task, a Writing task and a Listening task. They are not seen as examinations.

Keys and tapescripts

The following pages provide keys to all the exercises, and tapescripts of sections E and H.

Where no single answer is possible — for example, where students are asked to explain terms or interpret — this is signalled by 'No key is possible'. In general, there is no key for section F, which is exploited through questions etc. in section G.

The recording

The cassettes contain the texts of sections E (UNDERSTANDING A LECTURE) and H (UNDERSTANDING DISCOURSE). Introductions etc. by announcers have been cut to a minimum in order not to waste recording time. Similarly, pauses between lecture sections have been made deliberately short, since it is assumed that where necessary the teacher or student will stop the tape and possibly rewind it in order to listen for a second time.

UNIT 1: EPIDEMIOLOGY (1)

A. Understanding a printed text (1)

KEY

1 As 'a state of complete physical, mental and social well-being and not merely the absence of disease or infirmity'.
2 From health to terminal illness.
3 72%
4 Patients dying.
5 2,500

B. Check your understanding

KEY

1 No.
2 Few.
3 Treat themselves or seek help from a neighbour or a chemist.
4 64%
5 Respiratory illnesses and mental disturbances.
6 In the early stages.
7 Patients with serious illnesses or whose illness is difficult to diagnose.
8 Four or five.
9 Lung cancer.
10 A high-risk category.

C. Increase your vocabulary

KEY

1
- easy
- complete
- merely
- quantify
- truly

2
- people
- illnesses

3

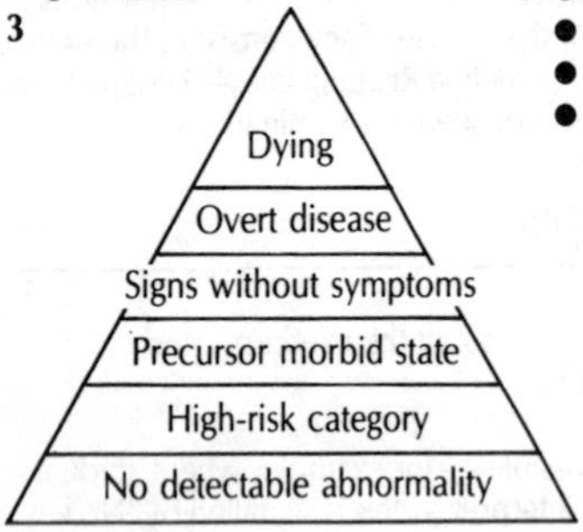

Dying
Overt disease
Signs without symptoms
Precursor morbid state
High-risk category
No detectable abnormality

4
- the majority
- regarded as
- for example
- given rise to
- undetected

5
- No key is possible.

6
- synonymous
- community
- impairment
- population

D. Check your grammar

KEY

1

work	is called
concentrate	is
are	refers
are seen	is examined
feels	gives
consults	is treated

2
- In 1939, Chain and Florey undertook an investigation of antibiotics.
- This discovery was made by accident.
- Fleming discovered penicillin in 1928.
- He put it aside as a curiosity.
- Penicillin is a fungus which was found to kill bacteria.
- They described the properties of penicillin in mice.
- Fleming failed to recognise the potential of penicillin.
- Because of the war, production was transferred to the USA.
- Penicillin made in the USA was used to treat casualties in the last years of the war.
- Penicillin was first given to humans in Oxford in 1941.

3 Fleming discovered penicillin in 1928. This discovery was made by accident. Penicillin is a fungus which was found to kill bacteria. Fleming failed to recognise the potential of penicillin. He put it aside as a curiosity. In 1939, Chain and Florey undertook an investigation of antibiotics. They described the properties of penicillin in mice. Penicillin was first given to humans in Oxford in 1941. Production was transferred to the USA because of the war. Penicillin made in the USA was used to treat casualties in the last years of the war.

E. Understanding a lecture

TAPESCRIPT

You are now going to hear part of a lecture. The lecture will be divided into short sections to help you understand it. Here is the first section. Are you ready?

Hello! In this lecture, we are going to look at what we mean by illness and disease. You might think that illness and disease are synonymous, that is, that they mean the same thing. But that's not quite true. Let me explain the difference. Illness is the experience of feeling unwell: it is the feeling of ill-health that often accompanies disease. Disease is a disturbance of the structure or function of part of the body, for instance by cancer or infection with micro-organisms. It is something that can usually be measured in some way or looked at under a microscope. But is this difference of any importance? And if so why? That's what we'll be considering today.

▶▶▶

When a person feels that something is wrong with part of their body, such as pain, weakness or nausea, this subjective complaint is called a symptom. That's spelt S–Y–M–P–T–O–M — symptom. When people feel ill, they complain of symptoms. But it is quite possible to have a disease and not feel ill at all. Does that sound complicated? Perhaps an example will make it clearer. Let's take the example of hypertension. You may not have heard that word before, so I'll spell it. H–Y–P–E–R–T–E–N–S–I–O–N — hypertension. It means high blood pressure. You can't feel it when you've got it, but it results in disease developing inside your body, particularly in your blood vessels. You can see the damage if you look at the back of someone's eye with a special instrument, which is called an ophthalmoscope — O–P–H–T–H–A–L–M–O–S–C–O–P–E. Ophthalmoscope.

▶▶▶

When a doctor finds something abnormal on examining a patient, this is called a clinical sign. S–I–G–N. Sign. So, a symptom is something the patient reports, and a sign is something the doctor may finds when examining the patient. When someone feels unwell, the doctor tries to find out what the problem is. This process is called diagnosis. D–I–A–G–N–O–S–I–S. Diagnosis. It involves asking the patient about his or her symptoms and examining the patient to look for signs. Each disease has a characteristic pattern of symptoms and signs. The doctor fits them into a pattern, like a jigsaw, and with luck finds the answer.

But if a person with a disease such as hypertension doesn't feel ill, how do they come to see a doctor? The answer is that often they don't until it's too late. By then, some catastrophe has occurred, such as a heart attack. You can't do much about such things when they've happened. But you can prevent them. For instance, everyone over a certain age can have their blood pressure measured every year, just in case. If it's too high, they can take tablets to make it lower. Prevention is much better than cure. It is fairly cheap, whereas modern technological treatment is too expensive for most countries to afford. And cures are rare, except with infectious diseases. Did you think medicine in the developed world was about curing people? I'm afraid that's rather an idealistic notion. Much of medicine is descriptive or palliative. You can remove people's symptoms. If you are lucky, you can stop the disease getting worse. But you can't often get rid of it completely.

KEY

Section 1 ————————————————————
● illness and disease
● cancer, infection with micro-organisms

Section 2 ————————————————————
● high blood pressure
● ophthalmoscope

Section 3 ————————————————————
● a clinical sign
● diagnosis

Section 4 ————————————————————
● prevention
● infectious disease

G. Check your understanding

KEY
1 ● No key is possible.
2 ● epidemiology
  ● infant mortality rate
  ● standardised mortality rate
3 ● incorrect   ● incorrect
  ● correct   ● incorrect
  ● incorrect   ● correct
  ● correct   ● incorrect
  ● correct   ● correct

H. Understanding discourse

TAPESCRIPT
You are now going to hear two people talking. The first speaker is trying to find out how to use a public telephone.

A Excuse me. Could you help me please?

B Certainly. If I can. What's the problem?

A I want to make a telephone call. But I don't understand how the pay telephone works.

B That's easy. Let me explain. First of all, you lift the handset. You'll hear the dialling tone and see a flashing light, saying 'Insert money'. Do you follow me so far?

A Not really. Could you speak more slowly please?

B I'm sorry. Of course. The part of the telephone that you speak into is called the handset. Here it is. You lift it up and put it to your ear. Try it. Can you hear a noise?

A No I can't. I can't hear anything at all.

B That means the telephone is broken. Here! Let's try the next one. Can you hear the tone? Listen!

A Yes, this one seems to be working. What do I do next?

B Can you see the flashing light? What does it say?

A It says 'Insert money'. Does that mean I have to put some money in?

B Yes.

A How much do I put in?

B It depends where you want to ring to. The minimum charge is ten pence. Have you got ten pence?

A I think so. Here we are. I'll put it in.

B Now you dial the number by pushing the buttons.

A What sound will it make?

B If it is ringing, you will hear two short tones repeated every few seconds. If the line is engaged, you will hear a longer single tone repeated.

A I'm afraid I don't quite follow that. What does this tone mean?

B That means it's ringing.

A Good. Thank you very much for your help.

A Not at all.

KEY
1 No precise key possible. The main points are: Lift up the handset. Listen for the dialling tone. Insert money. Dial the number.
2 ● Excuse me
  ● 'Insert money'
  ● ten pence
  ● two short tones repeated every few seconds

KING'S College LONDON *Founded* 1829

UNIT 2: EPIDEMIOLOGY (2)

A. Understanding a printed text (1)

1 Four and a half billion patients in the practice
  Half the practice are villagers
  Trade, aid, arms and energy.
2 Gross national product.
3 24th
4 About 800 million.
5 A million dollars a minute/$450 billion each year.

B. Check your understanding

1 4.6 billion.
2 2 billion.
3 Three-quarters.
4 A condition of life so characterised by malnutrition, illiteracy, disease, high infant mortality and low life expectancy as to be beneath any reasonable definition of human decency.
5 More than 30 million.
6 Those in towns.
7 Forty thousand.
8 20 billion US dollars.
9 Nuclear arsenals.
10 50 acres a minute.

C. Increase your vocabulary

1 ● doubled
  ● more
  ● poorest
  ● end
  ● exporter
2 ● injustice
  ● about
  ● shows
  ● remain
  ● absolute
  ● care for
3 No key is possible.

4 ● three-quarters
  ● expenditure
  ● access
  ● slum
  ● sanitation
5 No key is possible.
6 ● improved
  ● relieving
  ● requires
  ● benefit
  ● reduce

D. Check your grammar

1 ● You must work hard, if you want to become a doctor.
  ● If you don't study, you won't learn anything.
  ● If they are rich, they'll be able to get health care.
  ● If you are ill, you need to see a doctor.
  ● If money is spent on arms, there is less to spend on health and education.
  ● You can improve the health of the poor, if you relieve their poverty.
  ● If she falls over, she'll hurt herself.
  ● If it rains, the plants will grow.
  ● You'll get very tired, if you don't sleep.
  ● If he breaks his leg, he will need to go to hospital.
2 No key is possible.
3 No key is possible.

E. Understanding a lecture

You are now going to listen to a lecture. The lecture will be divided into short sections to help you understand it. Are you ready? Here is the first section.

Good morning! In today's lecture, I'm going to talk about measuring things in medicine. This is very important, particularly in epidemiology. You have to be able to describe things exactly, if you want to know how common an illness is, or to work out when it occurs. Otherwise, what you say will have little meaning. In order to describe things exactly, you give them a numerical value. That means, you express them in numbers. Expressing facts in numbers is known as statistics. Let's look at this a little more closely.

▶▶▶

If I said that many people in England and Wales die from heart disease, it would be true. You might even find it interesting. But it would be inexact. You wouldn't know, for instance, whether most people who die in England and Wales die from heart disease, or only a small proportion. If I had told you that 155,647 people had died from heart disease in England and Wales in 1979, that would have been more helpful. You would have had an exact measure of the number that died, and you would know the length of time in which they died. But you still wouldn't have an exact description of the problem. In fact, in 1979, the number of people who died in England and Wales from all causes was 593,019. So now we can work out what proportion of deaths was due to heart disease. It was 155,647 out of 593,019. If you use your pocket calculator, this comes out as 26.3% or just over a quarter. Rates are more usually expressed in numbers per 1000, so our numbers become a rate of 263 per 1000 deaths. But it's actually more useful to express death rates in terms of living people rather than dead people. In fact, if we look up the number of people dying from heart attacks, it was 220.18 per 100,000 of the population in England and Wales in 1979.

▶▶▶

At this point, I'd better introduce you to terms that you are often going to meet in reading about medicine. The first of these terms is incidence. That's spelt I–N–C–I–D–E–N–C–E. Incidence. The incidence of a disease is the rate of occurrence of new cases. In other words, it's the number of new cases of a disease, divided by the total population at risk, per unit time. Does that sound difficult to understand? It's the sort of thing you have to write down and look at to understand properly. Now I'll confuse you even more by telling you about the second term, prevalence. That's spelt P–R–E–V–A–L–E–N–C–E. Prevalence. The prevalence of a disease is the total number of persons with the disease in the population. In other words, prevalence is the total number of existing cases divided by the total population. The incidence is usually smaller than the prevalence, because the incidence only measures new cases, whereas the prevalence measures all cases, both new and old.

▶▶▶

So, statistics are very important in medicine. But don't get the idea that they tell you everything. As an anonymous Frenchman remarked: 'Statistics are like bikinis: they give an idea, but hide the essential.' Let me give you an example. If I told you that the average life expectancy in developing countries in the 1960s was 49, you might assume that everyone died at about the age of 49. In fact, because many died in infancy, the life expectancy of those surviving childhood was considerably longer than 49. Of course, there are other statistical methods which would express this problem more accurately. But we've run out of time in this lecture, so they'll have to wait for another day.

KEY

Section 1
- measuring things in medicine
- statistics

Section 2

	No. of deaths in the year 1979 in England and Wales
Heart disease	155,647
Total	593,019

∴
- proportion of deaths from heart disease = 26.3%
- rate of deaths from heart disease = 263 per 1000
- rate of death from heart attacks in the total population = 220.18 per 100,000

Section 3

$$\text{Incidence} = \frac{\text{new cases of disease}}{\text{total population at risk}} \text{ per unit time}$$

$$\text{Prevalence} = \frac{\text{total number of existing cases}}{\text{total population}}$$

Section 4
- they give an idea, but hide the essential
- because many die in infancy

G. Check your understanding

KEY

1
- pace
- mankind
- association
- decline
- disguise
2 No key is possible.
3
- correct
- incorrect

- correct
- incorrect
- incorrect
- incorrect
- correct
- incorrect
- incorrect
- incorrect
- incorrect

4 Written summary.
   This could equally well be used as an oral exercise in class. Students could be asked what they saw as the main points in the passage. This might lead on to a discussion of what information is very important and what is only additional to the main facts. Reducing each paragraph to essential detail might be practised before students are asked to write anything by themselves. The notes in the margins may be helpful.

H. Understanding discourse

TAPESCRIPT
On your tape you will hear a conversation between two students. One is new to the medical school and the other is explaining the location of various departments to him.

A: When I arrive at the medical school, where do I go?
B: Are you going by car?
A: Yes, I am.
B: In that case, you should go through the back entrance in St Charles Street. On your left, you will see the car park, and to your right the Physiology block. Straight ahead is the Biochemistry block. From the car park, walk between the Biochemistry and Physiology blocks and then turn left. In front of you, you will see the Students' Residence. To the right of you will be the Pharmacology block.
A: Whereabouts are the administration offices?
B: They are on the first floor of the Students' Residence.
A: And the canteen?
B: That's on the ground floor of the residence.
A: Perhaps I should go by bus and leave the car at home.
B: Well, there's a bus stop just outside the main entrance to the college.
A: How do I find my way from the main entrance to the Students' Residence?
B: As you go through the main gate, there's a lawn on your left, with trees beyond it, in front of the Physiology block. On your right is a small gate house. If you go straight on, past the Anatomy and Pharmacology blocks, you'll come to the residence. D'you think you'll remember all that?
A: I doubt it! I think I'd better write it down. Now . . .

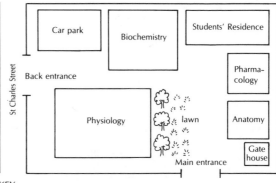

KEY

1 the back gate
2 on the first floor of the Students' Residence
3 on the ground floor of the residence
4 trees
5 just outside the main entrance

UNIT 3: MALNUTRITION

A. Understanding a printed text (1)

KEY
1 Malnutrition of affluent societies.
2 Overnutrition and obesity.
3 Definition, epidemiology, aetiological factors, associated diseases.
4 Paragraph 7. Disorders associated with obesity.

B. Check your understanding

KEY
1 Those who have 'thrifty' metabolism.
2 Obesity, faster growth, earlier puberty, greater fertility and earlier aging.
3 W/H^2 where W is the weight in kg and H is the height in metres.
4 Because most of their fat contemporaries have already died.

5 Commoner in the lower socio-economic classes.
6 Less refined foods and more fresh foods.
7 In preparation for the demands of breast feeding.
8 Ischaemic heart disease and cerebrovascular disease.
9 1%
10 They cannot dress smartly or fashionably.

C. Increase your vocabulary

KEY
1 ● virtually
  ● affluent
  ● thrifty
  ● surplus
  ● susceptible
2 ● synthesis
  ● secretion
  ● resistance and tolerance
  ● tendency
  ● neoplasm

3 ● intake
  ● impaired
  ● unfortunately
  ● malignant
4 No key is possible.
5 ● index
  ● syntheses
6 ● aggravates
  ● prone to
  ● especially
  ● hazardous
  ● hinders

D. Check your grammar

KEY
1 (a) a/–/the/the/–
  (b) a/a/the/a/–/the/–
  (c) the/the/a/–
  (d) the/–/an/–
  (e) the/an/the
2 (a) nevertheless
  (b) however
  (c) although
  (d) however
  (e) whereas
3 (a) The operation was performed by a group of Japanese surgeons.
  (b) The double-helix model of DNA was proposed by Watson and Crick, while the alpha-helix of giant protein molecules was described by Pauling.
  (c) The layout of bases, sugars and phosphates within the molecules was discovered during the 1930s and 1940s.
  (d) The atom can be split into smaller particles such as protons, electrons and neutrons.
  (e) The presence of obesity can be ascertained from an examination of the patient, but a weighing machine or scales is needed to measure their weight accurately.

E. Understanding a lecture

TAPESCRIPT

Listen to this lecture which is about chemical terminology and the composition of foodstuffs. As you listen, look at the table given in your book. Then fill in the missing data.

Good morning, ladies and gentlemen. You've been reading about problems of nutrition, and considering some aspects of the relationship between dietary habits and disease. Before we look into this any further, we must refresh our memories about the chemical constituents of food and make sure that we are familiar with basic chemical terminology. I shall call this lecture 'the macromolecules of life'.

▶▶▶

I mentioned the word 'macromolecules'. What does this mean? 'Macro' simply means large. And I expect you remember what a molecule is. It is the structure formed when two atoms become bound together. Atoms are the smallest possible particles of an element. The hundred or so elements in nature are substances which can't be split into simpler substances by chemical means. The atom, of course, is itself composed of smaller particles. But these are the concern of subatomic physics, not biochemistry. A further term of which we should remind ourselves is compound. A compound is a substance made by the chemical combination of two or more elements.

The elements are represented by symbols, C for carbon, H for hydrogen, N for nitrogen and so on. Compounds can be represented in two ways. Firstly by writing the letters of the constituents down in formulae. If you look at the table of frequently occurring organic groupings in your book, you will see for instance that the grouping carbon-oxygen-oxygen-hydrogen is represented as $-COOH$; this is known as an acid. Similarly an alcohol is denoted by the formula, CH_2OH. The second way of representing molecules is by drawing expanded formulae, which are two-dimensional pictures. The elements are joined together by lines, each line representing a chemical bond. Each atom of an element can make a certain number of bonds with other atoms: the number for each type of atom is constant and is known as its valency. Hydrogen, for instance, has a valency of one, and carbon has a valency of four. The atoms may be joined together in branching rows and also in rings. At the bottom of the table, you can see a drawing of a benzene ring, that's spelt B–E–N–Z–E–N–E. Of course, molecules in living systems are often very large, and can be folded round in complex three-dimensional structures. A well-known example is that of deoxyribonucleic acid or DNA. This is the substance in the nucleus of every cell which contains the genetic code which determines how an organism grows or develops. It takes the form of a double helix.

▶▶▶

The three main types of macromolecule in foodstuffs are proteins, carbohydrates and fats. Proteins are made up of smaller molecules called amino acids, which are given this name because they contain both amino and acid groups. Proteins form the main structures of human cells. They are found in meat and in some plant foodstuffs such as beans. The second main group of macromolecules are called carbohydrates. These are made up of smaller molecules called sugars. They are found mainly in plants especially in so-called starchy foods like cereals or root vegetables. The third main type of macromolecule is fats, which are composed of chains of fatty acids. Fats are also sometimes known as lipids. L–I–P–I–D–S.

▶▶▶

When food is digested, the macromolecules are broken down into their constituent molecules and absorbed as such. Amino acids are used to form protein in cells. Sugars are broken down to form energy in a process called glycolysis. Fats provide a way of storing surplus food intake, and they can be converted into the sugar, glucose, in the liver in a process known as gluconeogenesis. Sugars can also be converted into fats. If too much fat or carbohydrate is eaten regularly, obesity may result. If not enough food is eaten to provide energy, the body will first of all use up its stores of fat. When these are exhausted, it will begin to break down the structural protein of which the tissues are composed. For amino acids can be used to create energy too. The individual may slowly waste away. You will be going on to consider the effects of starvation very soon.

KEY
Section 1───────────
● the macromolecules of life

Section 2

- two atoms become bound together
- an element
- can't be split into simpler substances
- the chemical combination of two or more elements

Section 3

- CH_2OH; acid; benzene
- a double helix

Section 4

- proteins, carbohydrates and fats
- smaller molecules called amino acids
- smaller molecules called sugars
- chains of fatty acids
- lipids

Section 5

- to form protein in cells
- broken down to form energy
- converted into the sugar, glucose, in the liver
- begin to break down the structural protein of which the tissues are composed.

TABLE 1. *Frequently occurring organic groupings*

Formula	Name	Expanded formula
.CH₃	Methyl	
.CH₂.CH₃	Ethyl	
.C:C.	Double bond	
.CHO	Aldehyde	
.CH₂OH	Alcohol	
.CO	Ketone	
.COOH	Acid	
.CH₂NH₂	Amine	
	Benzene ring	

G. Check your understanding

KEY

1
1. crop failures, droughts, overpopulation, poverty and civil strife
2. fat
3. protein
4. 150g
5. 25 per cent
6. the brain
7. because the heart can shrink to half or even a third of its normal weight
8. it can become paper thin and almost transparent
9. keto acids
10. because it reduces the need for gluconeogenesis and so spares protein breakdown in the liver
11. due to loss of elasticity of the connective tissue and to a fall in serum albumin
12. starvation of babies
13. 'protein-energy malnutrition'; 'first-second'.
14. between 9 months and 2 years
15. 5 million
16. because they increase the need for protein and so worsen the deficiency
17. the brain
18. education in good agriculture and good nutrition

2 The comparison of starvation and kwashiorkor can be made as an oral class exercise if this is thought useful. The differences are readily evident in the text. Kwashiorkor involves protein deficiency and occurs in small children, whereas starvation involves deficiency of fat, carbohydrate and protein and may occur at any age.

3 It is advisable to go through the students' answers to question 2 above, before a written account is attempted.

H. Understanding discourse

TAPESCRIPT

You are now going to hear a conversation between two students about the course at their medical school.

Student A: How many students are there in the medical school? It all seems much bigger than what I've been used to.

Student B: There are about eighty in each year. The course lasts five years. So there are about 400.

Student A: And what happens in each of those five years? I don't really understand what the course involves.

Student B: Well, I'll try and give you a rough idea. The course is split into two parts. There's the pre-clinical course, which lasts two years. That's followed by the clinical course, which lasts three years.

Student A: I'm just starting the pre-clinical course. The timetable seems full up with lectures and practical work in laboratories.

Student B: That's right. You don't actually spend much time with patients until the clinical course. You spend nearly all your time in the medical school.

Student A: I see that I'm going to study anatomy, physiology and biochemistry. Is there anything else?

Student B: Yes. You'll have some lectures on statistics, sociology and psychology. And you'll learn a lot of pharmacology.

Student A: And what about exams?

Student B: Your main exams will be at the end of the pre-clinical course. You'll have to write essays and do multiple choice questions. You'll also have oral exams, where you answer questions face to face with the examiner.

Student A: I'm not looking forward to that. Still, it's a long way off. And what about you? What are you doing?

Student B: I'm coming to the end of the clinical course.

Student A: I'm not quite sure what that consists of.

Student B: Well, you spend most of your time in the hospital itself. You get lectures, but not as many as in the pre-clinical course. You're attached to doctors, who teach you about the patients they are looking after.

Student A: And what subjects do you actually study?

7

Student B: A bit of everything really. But the exams at the end are in medicine, surgery, obstetrics and gynaecology, pathology and therapeutics.

Student A: It sounds an awful lot.

Student B: It is. You have to study hard and learn large numbers of facts.

Student A: And if you pass your final exams? I'm not really clear what happens next.

Student B: They you start as a doctor on the wards. And that's when the real learning begins.

UNIT 4: BIOCHEMISTRY

A. Understanding a printed text (1)

KEY

1 The study of the molecular basis of life.
2 The chemical bases of many central processes are now understood. It is now known that common molecular patterns and principles underlie the diverse expressions of life. Biochemistry is profoundly influencing medicine.
3 Its polarity and cohesiveness.
4 80
5 It attenuates them.

B. Check your understanding

KEY

1   1 DNA, RNA, protein.
   2 Adenosine triphosphate.
   3 The diagnosis of genetic disorders, infectious diseases and cancers.
   4 Insulin, growth hormone.
   5 Triangular.
   6 Polar molecules.
   7 A highly regular crystalline structure.
   8 3.4.
   9 Polar molecules.
   10 By creating water-free micro-environments where polar interactions have maximal strength.
2 ● incorrect   ● incorrect
● correct   ● correct
● incorrect
3 Water diminishes the strength of electrostatic attractions.
Electrostatic attractions between ions are markedly weakened by the presence of water.
Water attenuates electrostatic attractions between charged groups.
4 No key is possible.

C. Increase your vocabulary

KEY

1 discovery, elucidation, determination, unraveling
2 ● diverse   ● reveal
● profoundly   ● valuable
● indispensable   ● rational

3 ● ion   4 nuclei
● gene   5 ● attraction
● catalyst   ● constant
● vacuum   ● capacity
● solvent   ● oriented
● serum   ● diffuse

D. Check your grammar

KEY

1 ● is composed of   ● spending
● consists of   ● learning
● contain   ● functioning
● is comprised of   ● to create
● is composed of   ● to apply
● consists of, contains 3 ● but
2 ● to study   ● when
● to take place   ● and
● developing   ● because
● eating   ● before
● to appreciate

E. Understanding a lecture

TAPESCRIPT

Good morning everyone!
You've been considering aspects of the chemical basis of life. But what in fact is the human body composed of? We know that it contains complex macromolecules. But let us consider in what proportions these are present. The body can also be considered in terms of liquid and solid, and in terms of percentages of the different elements present. Today, we shall examine this in detail. We will then go on to look at the structure of a typical cell.

▶▶▶

Let's start with the macromolecules. Exact proportions of these in the body will vary. Muscular people will have a greater proportion of protein and obese people a greater proportion of lipids. In general, protein accounts for between 15 per cent and 20 per cent of body weight. Lipids may account for anything from 3 per cent to 20 per cent. Carbohydrates may account for between 1 per cent and 15 per cent of body weight. There are also small organic molecules and inorganic molecules. Each of these groups forms about 1 per cent of body weight. As you can see, these percentage figures do not add up to one hundred. That is because they concern only the solid matter in the body. But the total solid matter in the body comprises only between 20 per cent and 40 per cent of the total weight. The rest is, quite simply, water.

▶▶▶

But what then of the elements? You may ask how one can possibly work out the elemental contents of the body. In fact, this is comparatively simple to do. The body is incinerated and a variety of techniques used to separate out all the individual elements. All that is needed then is a balance. A large part of the body is composed of oxygen, carbon and hydrogen. Oxygen accounts for 65 per cent of body weight, carbon for 19 per cent, and hydrogen for 10 per cent. The fact that most of the body is water accounts for much of the oxygen and hydrogen. Then there are the elements of nitrogen, calcium and phosphorus, which represent 3 per cent, 2 per cent and 1.1 per cent respectively. Most of the phosphorus and calcium is combined as calcium phosphate, which forms bone. There are small amounts of potassium, sulphur, sodium and chlorine in the body. Together they account for 0.9 per cent of body weight. There are also traces of various metals.

▶▶▶

Now turn to the diagram in your books. This represents the structure of a typical animal cell. I'm sure you are all familiar with the details, but frequent revision is always a good idea in the study of medical sciences. The study of cells and their structure is known as cytology — that's spelt C–Y–T–O–L–O–G–Y — whereas the study of the structure of tissues is known as histology — H–I–S–T–O–L–O–G–Y. Cells have a number of complex sub-units and these are known as organelles — I'll spell that out for you, too — O–R–G–A–N–E–L–L–E–S. On your diagram, the coating of a cell is known as the membrane. The large grey area in the centre is the nucleus. This contains all the cell DNA. Much of this is concentrated in the nucleolus — N–U–C–L–E–O–L–U–S — which is represented by the black dot in the figure. The nucleus is surrounded by a membrane in which there are gaps, known as pores. The nuclear membrane is connected with the cell membrane by a labyrinth of membrane called the endoplasmic reticulum — that's spelt E–N–D–O–P–L–A–S–M–I–C — endoplasmic — R–E–T–I–C–U–L–U–M — reticulum. This is studded with ribosomes — R–I–B–O–S–O–M–E–S — in which protein synthesis takes place. Then there are the mitochondria — M–I–T–O–C–H–O–N–D–R–I–A — which are perhaps the most interesting of the organelles from a biochemical point of view. For it is in the mitochondria that the citric acid cycle takes place. You will be refreshing your memories about the citric acid cycle and glycolysis in my next lecture.

KEY

1 The composition of the human body by weight

	Substance	% body weight
Types of molecule	protein	15–20
	lipid	3–20
	carbohydrate	1–15
	small organic molecules	1
	inorganic molecules	1
Water/solid	water	60–80
	solid	20–40
Elements	oxygen	65
	carbon	18
	hydrogen	10
	nitrogen	3
	calcium	2
	phosphorus	1.1
	potassium	
	sulphur	0.9
	sodium	
	chlorine	
	various metals	traces

2 Schematic diagram of a 'typical' animal cell

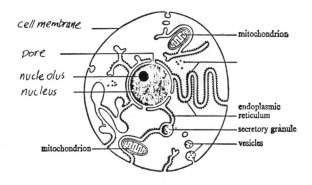

3 ● the fact that most of the body is water
● cytology is the study of cells, whereas histology is the study of tissues
● in the nucleus
● in the ribosomes
● the citric acid cycle

G. Check your understanding

KEY

1 1 Reversible ones.
  2 Electrostatic bonds, hydrogen bonds and van der Waals bonds.
  3 Coulomb's law $F = \dfrac{q^1 q^2}{r^2 D}$, where q^1 and q^2 are the charges of the two groups, r is the distance between them, and D is the dielectric constant of the medium.
  4 Ionic bond, salt linkage, salt bridge, ion pair.
  5 Hydrogen bond.
  6 Donors and acceptors are oxygen or nitrogen, but the donors differ in having a covalently attached hydrogen atom.
  7 Covalent; hydrogen; van der Waals.
  8 Protein, DNA.
  9 They repeal each other.
  10 Oxygen

2 No specific key can be given. The text states that the three bonds differ in geometry, strength and specificity and are affected in different ways by the presence of water. The main points are as follows. Electrostatic bonds occur between two groups with opposite electrical charges. In hydrogen bonds, the molecules need not be charged. They bond by sharing a hydrogen atom. Van der Waals bonds are the result of a weaker non-specific attraction between two molecules whose electric charge distribution is not perfectly symmetrical.

H. Understanding discourse

TAPESCRIPT
Listen to this conversation. A student is asking his tutor some questions about the breakdown of glucose to form energy.

Tutor: Yes, Ahmed. What can I do for you?
Pupil: I'm afraid I found your lecture on the glycolytic pathway difficult to follow. It all seems so complicated.
Tutor: It is complicated, but it is very logical. Do you understand what glycolysis is?
Pupil: Yes, I think so. It means the breakdown of glucose to pyruvic acid.

Tutor: That's right. It's part of a metabolic pathway that takes place in cells. Glucose from the blood-stream is broken down in a series of ten chemical reactions, releasing energy.

Pupil: But what I don't understand is where oxygen comes in. Don't you need oxygen to create energy?

Tutor: Yes, you are partly right. Oxygen is essential in the breakdown of glucose to carbon dioxide and water, which releases energy. But that process is separated into two pathways. The glycolytic pathway is only the first of these. Glycolysis takes place without oxygen. The glucose, as you told me, is only broken down as far as pyruvic acid. Can you think what might happen next?

Pupil: No. Not really.

Tutor: Well, the second pathway involved in the breakdown of glucose is called the citric acid cycle. It is called a cycle because there is a circular chain of eight reactions. These were discovered by Hans Krebs. The pyruvic acid feeds into the cycle. It is broken down to carbon dioxide and water, and much energy is produced. The citric acid cycle can only take place in the presence of oxygen.

Pupil: And what happens if there is no oxygen?

Tutor: Well, pyruvic acid can be converted to lactic acid. That releases some energy. But the cell can't function if much lactic acid is present. So the whole process would soon stop if there were no oxygen.

Pupil: And in what form is the energy produced?

Tutor: That's quite simple really. Of course, energy isn't something that exists freely. It can exist in the form, for instance, of heat or light. In biochemical systems, energy is produced in a chemical form. The energy released in the breakdown of glucose is put into a particular molecule. The energy is used to join a molecule called ADP to an extra phosphate group to form the molecule known as ATP. The ATP is in effect an energy carrier. It will easily give up its energy to be used in other chemical reactions. In all, thirty-eight molecules of ATP are produced during the breakdown of one molecule of glucose to carbon dioxide and water. Does that make it any clearer?

Pupil: Yes. Thank you very much. If I look it up again in the textbook, I think I shall understand it this time.

KEY

1 1. pyruvic acid
2. glycolysis
3. ten
4. lactic acid
5. citric acid cycle
6. eight
7. carbon dioxide and water
8. thirty-eight

2 ● the citric acid cycle
● because the cell can't function if much lactic acid is present
● a molecule of ADP and a phosphate group

UNIT 5: DRUG ABUSE

A. Understanding a printed text (1)

KEY
1 Fermentation.
2 More than 2000 years BC.
3 To achieve states of ecstasy or frenzy.
4 Islam.
5 Ethiopia and the Yemen.

B. Check your understanding

KEY
1 1. Yeasts.
2. It was used in medicine and religion.
3. Drunkenness amongst priests.
4. Devout Buddhists, Hindu Brahmins, Muslims, some Protestant sects.
5. Religious tenet.
6. Because they did not discover the secret of fermentation.
7. Opium poppy, Indian hemp, tobacco plant, coffee plant, tea bush, cocoa plant, peyote cactus.
8. No.

2 No key is possible. This is intended as an exercise in distilling the important points from a detailed passage written in elaborate English. A standard answer might run as follows:

Humanity has a striking capacity for finding and using psychoactive drugs. No other species behaves in this way, although animals can be made dependent on drugs under laboratory conditions. Equally striking are the strong feelings in human societies about psychoactive substances. Drugs are praised for their pleasurable effects. They are condemned for causing dependence and for their harmful medical and social effects.

C. Increase your vocabulary

KEY
1 ● readily
● to facilitate
● exposed
● to convert
● intoxicating
2 ● beverages
● requisite
● prominent
● proscribe
● abortive
● fundamental

3 No key is possible.
4 ● regulation
● ensurance
● enablement
● equation
● control
● containment
● generation
● exposure
5 No key is possible.

D. Check your grammar

KEY
1 ● extremely
● occasionally
● excessive
● easy
● successfully
● usually; newly
● adequate, potential
● commonly; careful

2 ● as/since
● as a result of
● as/since
● because of
● because
● for reasons of

E. Understanding a lecture

TAPESCRIPT

You will now hear a lecture. As you listen, try and take notes along the lines suggested in your textbook. You may have to listen more than once in order to pick out all the important points.

Drug abuse is an area in which terminology can be confusing. Terms are often used in a way which implies moral judgement. And people often mix up the questions of whether a drug is harmful and whether or not it is illegal. The potential harm of a drug is of course something that does not change. But legality and the way the drug is seen by society may vary widely. It is a curious fact that some societies have at times allowed the free use of drugs which at other times or in other societies have been considered so dangerous as to require the strictest forms of legal control.

▶▶▶

By the term abuse, we don't simply mean use. We mean that the drug is being used to a degree which causes either physical harm to the user or damage to his relationships or to those around him. Nor is abuse the same thing as dependence. By dependence, we mean that the user cannot do without the drug. This includes psychological dependence where the drug is regarded as an indispensable prop in the user's life and he is consequently not motivated to stop using it. But the main form of dependence with which we are concerned is true physical addiction. This is due to a direct chemical effect of the drug on the body. If the person stops taking the drug, very unpleasant and sometimes dangerous withdrawal effects occur. But, as I mentioned, addiction or dependence is not the same thing as abuse. Some drugs can be abused, but are not addictive.

▶▶▶

But what about the legality of drugs? How is that related to abuse? Well, drugs can only be widely abused if they are freely available. What do you think is the greatest drug abuse problem in Britain? Do you think it might be heroin or cocaine, or some other exotic compound that makes headlines in the press? No. In fact the most serious problem of abuse is with alcohol. This causes a huge amount of death, disease, crime, family break-up and economic loss to the country. Second comes tobacco which is legal, but causes the deaths of 100,000 people in Britain every year, as well as enormous costs to the National Health Service and to the economy in terms of working days lost. The third most important drugs of abuse are medically prescribed minor tranquillisers. Like alcohol and tobacco, these are addictive.

▶▶▶

Which other drugs are addictive? And is the addictive potential of a drug related to its ability to do harm to the body? In other words, are the most addictive drugs the most physically harmful? Probably the most addictive drug of all is heroin. But, in fact, heroin does not harm the body directly. The physical dangers of its use are related to the way in which it is used. Because supplies are illegal, exact doses cannot be ensured, and overdoses kill. The heroin is often adulterated with substances which are poisonous, and people sharing needles risk catching hepatitis B or AIDS. The main damage from heroin is social. People's whole way of life may be changed by the drug. The desire to obtain more is so strong that people will cheat or steal to get money to buy it with. Curiously, heroin withdrawal is not particularly dangerous. By contrast, untreated alcohol withdrawal has a mortality of fifteen per cent. Apart from opiates, the only illegal drugs in Britain which are physically addictive are barbiturates, which started as commonly prescribed

sleeping pills. The other main illegal drugs of abuse are amphetamines, cocaine, hallucinogens such as LSD, and marihuana. While each of these has its dangers, physical addiction is not one of them.

▶▶▶

You'll have gathered by now that the relation between drug abuse and legality in Britain is profoundly illogical. Why is this so? Well, it's obviously a product of historical circumstance. But the main factors perpetuating the situation are financial. The government receives huge amounts of money from the taxation of alcohol and cigarettes which it does not wish to lose. And the producers of alcohol and tobacco are powerful companies with political influence. The government thus has a strong financial interest in perpetuating the poisoning of its citizens. Of course, the only rational approach to drugs in society would be to limit access to all of them. Some people would argue that most drugs can be used sensibly without abuse, and that abuse simply reflects a defect in the individual's personality. Some would argue that each person should have the freedom to harm himself in any way that he pleases. The obvious reply is that individual freedom must be limited when it interferes with the general good or the fabric of society. But here we enter the realm of political philosophy. That's a topic for another day.

KEY
1 ● Abuse = use of a drug to a degree which causes physical harm to the user or damages his relationships or those around him.
  ● Dependence = the user cannot do without the drug.
  ● Two types of dependence: 1. psychological; 2. physical addiction
  ● Drugs causing the greatest problems of abuse in Britain:
    1. alcohol
    2. tobacco
    3. minor tranquillisers
  ● Dangers of heroin: overdose
                adulteration with poisons
                catching hepatitis B or AIDS from dirty needles
                social dangers — cheating and stealing
  ● Other physically addictive drugs illegal in Britain: barbiturates
  ● Drugs illegal but not physically addictive: amphetamines, cocaine, hallucinogens (e.g. LSD), marihuana.
2 ● withdrawal effects occur   ● social
  ● no   ● alcohol withdrawal
  ● 100,000
3 This is intended as an opportunity for class discussion. It could equally well be used as a topic for a short written essay.

G. Check your understanding

KEY
1 ● incorrect
  ● incorrect
  ● incorrect
  ● incorrect
  ● correct
  ● correct
2 No key is possible. (A typical answer might be as follows: Alcohol dependent drinkers are always problem drinkers. Most problem drinkers are heavy drinkers, but some are binge drinkers. Alcohol dependent drinkers are always heavy drinkers. Most heavy drinkers are not problem drinkers.)
3 No key is possible.

H. Understanding discourse

Doctor: Good morning, Mr Brown.
Brown: Good morning, doctor.
Doctor: What can I do for you today?
Brown: I'm not really sure, doctor. I'm having difficulty getting on with my wife, and I've been taking rather a lot of time off work recently. They're not very pleased with me. I feel I can't cope any more.
Doctor: Why have you been taking time off work?
Brown: Headaches, stomach aches, that sort of thing.
Doctor: Your breath smells of alcohol. Are you drinking a lot these days?
Brown: Oh, no. Not really, doctor. Drink's never been a problem with me.
Doctor: Have you ever felt you ought to cut down on your drinking?
Brown: No, I don't think so. I just enjoy a drink like lots of other people.

Doctor: Have people annoyed you by criticising your drinking?
Brown: Funny you should say that. My wife's always telling me to drink less. It makes me really angry.
Doctor: Have you ever felt bad or guilty about your drinking?
Brown: No. I haven't. Why should I?
Doctor: Have you ever had a drink first thing in the morning to get rid of a hangover?
Brown: Yes, of course. It's the best way, isn't it? It's what I call an 'eye-opener'.
Doctor: I think I'm beginning to get an idea of your problem, Mr Brown.

KEY
1 Mr Brown
2 He has been having difficulty getting on with his wife; he has taken a lot of time off work.
3 (i) Have you ever felt you ought to cut down on your drinking?
   (ii) Have people annoyed you by criticising your drinking?
   (iii) Have you ever felt bad or guilty about your drinking?
   (iv) Have you ever had a drink first thing in the morning to get rid of a hangover?
4 Yes.

CHECK YOUR PROGRESS (1)

A. Reading

KEY
The following are true:
1. b.
2. a. c. d.
3. a. c. e.
4. d. e.
5. b. c.
6. b. d. e.

B. Writing

It would be helpful to offer a selection of vocabulary that could be used in this exercise: e.g. *is caused by, occurs in, include, are said to be*, etc. Students should be encouraged to expand their descriptions as much as they can.

C. Listening

Today, we shall consider mechanisms of human heredity. This is important in medicine, because it is not only physical and intellectual characteristics that are influenced by heredity. Various forms of illness can also be transmitted from parent to child.

▶▶▶

All hereditary information is transmitted from parent to offspring through the inheritance of deoxyribonucleic acid or DNA. DNA codes for the production of ribonucleic acid or RNA. Through this, it determines protein synthesis. The DNA forms genes. A gene is a sequence of DNA which encodes for the amino acid sequence of a single polypeptide chain in a protein molecule. The amount of

DNA in each human cell is sufficient to make up more than 50,000 genes and so to specify more than 50,000 polypeptide chains. The genes are arranged in a linear sequence of DNA, which forms rod-shaped bodies known as chromosomes.

▶▶▶

Each human cell contains 46 chromosomes. Two of these concern the sex of the individual. These sex chromosomes are named X and Y. The female possesses two X chromosomes, whereas the male possesses one X chromosome and one Y chromosome. The remaining 44 chromosomes are non-sex chromosomes, also known as autosomes. There are in fact 22 pairs of these in each cell. They can be made visible under the microscope by special staining techniques.

▶▶▶

To understand how genetic information is passed on, we must look at what happens when cells divide. Of course, cells in the body are dividing all the time. And when the nuclei of such cells divide, the chromosome material is duplicated. In other words, both cells end up with a full set of chromosomes. This process is known as mitosis, M–I–T–O–S–I–S. But there is another sort of cell division which occurs in the formation of gametes in the ovary and testis. In this process, the number of chromosomes is reduced by half. The resulting cells each have half of the 22 pairs of autosomes and one of the sex chromosomes — in other words, 23 chromosomes in all. This type of division is known as meiosis, M–E–I–O–S–I–S. When the sperm and the egg combine, the resulting embryo has cells with 46 chromosomes, 23 from the father and 23 from the mother.

▶▶▶

Now, some individuals possess genes which are abnormal and so may lead to disease. These may be passed on to the offspring. For some conditions to appear, it is necessary that the individual possess a double dose of the abnormal gene, one from each parent. These are known as recessive conditions. An example of an autosomal recessive condition is sickle-cell anaemia. Usually both parents are normal because they each only possess one dose of the gene. They can each pass on either a normal or an abnormal gene to their offspring. Thus, chance dictates that an average one in four of their children will have a double dose of the abnormal gene and so be affected by the disease. Two in four of their children will have a single dose, and so not show the condition; but they can of course transmit the abnormal gene to their own offspring. One in four will have only the normal gene.

▶▶▶

In some conditions, only one dose of the abnormal gene is necessary for the disease to be expressed. Such genes are known as dominant. An example of an autosomal dominant disease is

Huntingdon's chorea. In dominant conditions, each affected individual will have an affected parent. On average, half the children of an affected individual will be affected.

KEY
The following are correct:
1. a. b. d.
2. d. e.
3. b. c. d.
4. b. e.
5. b. c.

UNIT 6: INFECTIOUS DISEASES

A. Understanding a printed text (1)

KEY
1 Improvements in sanitation, water supply and nutrition.
2 Diarrhoeal disease.
3 Climatic conditions, sanitation, the quality of the water supply, the specific disease resistance of the population at risk.
4 Reservoirs of infection and effective modes of transmission.
5 Human, animal and environment.
6 Airborne spread, spread by direct contact, spread by food and water.

B. Check your understanding

KEY
1 The following statements are true: b, d, g, j.
2 ● Tuberculosis.
  ● Immunodiagnosis.
  ● They may remain in the lymphatic circulation for many years.
  ● Infections which can be transmitted from animals to man.
  ● By aerosol from air-conditioning units.

C. Increase your vocabulary

KEY
1 A c.   ● affliction
  B d.   ● antibodies
  C e.   5 ● pathogen
  D b.   ● indigenous
  E a.   ● vary
2 spores, cysts, larvae, ova   ● viable
3 No key is possible.   ● contaminated
4 ● excrete   6 ● bacterium, protozoon
  ● eliminate   ● larvae
  ● vaccines

D. Check your grammar

KEY
1 No (precise) key is possible.
2 The nouns and definitions should be turned into sentences as shown in the examples. The correct pairings are Ab, Bd, Ce, Da, Ec.

E. Understanding a lecture

TAPESCRIPT
You will now hear part of a lecture on AIDS. Refer to the key words in your book and take notes as you listen.

Today, I am going to talk about the acquired immunodeficiency syndrome, popularly known as AIDS for short. AIDS is the end-stage of a chronic infection with a virus known as the human immunodeficiency virus or HIV. The virus slowly destroys the body's immune system.

▶▶▶

As far as the *history* of AIDS is concerned, it appears to be a new disease. It was first recognised in 1981 in the United States of America. The Centre for Diseases Control in Atlanta noted a surprisingly large number of cases of some extremely unusual diseases. One was Kaposi's sarcoma (or KS), a rare form of skin cancer. Another was pneumocystis carinii pneumonia or PCP, a rare lung infection. In normal circumstances, both these conditions were seen only in patients whose immune systems had been destroyed. But the new cases were all in previously healthy young people. And, curiously, ninety-two per cent of the cases involved homosexual men in three American cities. It was recognised that something new was happening, although the virus responsible for the disease was not isolated until 1983.

▶▶▶

The *transmission* of the human immunodeficiency virus is through blood or blood products. The most common methods of transmission are: firstly, through sexual activity, particularly anal intercourse; secondly, through the sharing of infected needles by those injecting drugs; and thirdly, through the accidental transfusion of patients in hospitals with infected blood. A fourth type of transmission which is becoming more common is the infection of unborn children by a mother who carries the virus. This is known as congenital infection.

▶▶▶

The *course* of the disease involves four stages as follows. Firstly, when the person becomes infected, they may feel generally unwell for a few days, as if they have a very bad cold. Afterwards, this disappears and they feel perfectly healthy; this is known as the asymptomatic stage. The person may continue to feel healthy for several years. The third stage is known as persistent generalised lymphadenopathy, or PGL for short. In PGL, most of the patient's lymph nodes swell up, but he still does not feel ill. The fourth stage is AIDS itself. Here, the patient suffers from unusual infections or tumours which the immune system is too weak to resist. The patient feels very unwell. After a period lasting months or even a year or two, the patient dies.

▶▶▶

The *prognosis* of the disease — that means the eventual outcome — is very poor. It is likely that everyone infected with HIV will eventually get AIDS. AIDS is thought to be fatal in all cases. There is no *treatment* for HIV infection. Nor has any method of preventing HIV infection been discovered.

KEY

1 It is necessary to master the art of taking abbreviated notes. An example would be as follows:
- *AIDS*. End stage HIV infection. Destroys immune system.
- *History*. New. Recognised 1981 USA. CDC Atlanta noticed cases rare diseases (KS & PCP). Usually found in immunosuppressed. Here healthy young. 92% male homosexuals from 3 US cities. Virus isolated 1983.
- *Transmission*. Blood/blood products. 1) sex, esp. anal. 2) infected needles. 3) transfusion. 4) congenital.
- *Course*. 4 stages: 1) When infected. Few days. Like bad cold. 2) Asymptomatic. May last years. 3) PGL. Nodes swell. Not ill. 4) AIDS. Unusual infections/tumours. Patient v. unwell. Death months/year or two.
- *Prognosis*. Poor. HIV→AIDS. Fatal. No treatment. No prevention.

2 It would be advisable to check the student's notes before he attempts to expand them. No key is possible.

G. Check your understanding

KEY

1 No exact key is possible.
- *Endemic* illness is regularly present in a particular population; *epidemic* illness is widespread in a population for a short time only.
- An *acute* illness comes sharply to a crisis whereas a *chronic* illness is continual and lasts a long time.
- *Susceptibility* is a state of being sensitive to or easily affected by an illness; *resistance* is the reverse.
- *Antibodies* are substances produced by the body's immune system to attack a particular foreign organism or substance, the latter being known as an *antigen*.

2 No key is possible.

3 1. Human immunoglobulin.
2. Attenuated live strains.
3. Immunosuppression by kwashiorkor, malignancies, steroids or cytotoxic drugs.
4. 14–16 months.
5. 3 days.
6. Encephalitis and SSPE.
7. It failed to raise antibody to the F protein. It caused a severe reaction at the site of the injection or a bizarre form of measles.
8. The severely immunocompromised.
9. Heat. Maternal antibody.
10. Annual mass vaccination of at least 90% of all susceptible children, or an on-going programme in which 75% of all susceptible children are vaccinated at 6 months of age.

H. Understanding discourse

TAPESCRIPT
Listen to the discussion. The teacher is asking the class about immunity and immunisation.

Teacher: Right! Can anyone explain to me what immunity is?
Student A: It means to be safe from something.
Teacher: And what does it mean when we're talking about infections?
Student A: It means that the body has defences against them.
Teacher: Yes, that's right. And how does it defend itself?
Student A: One way is with antibodies.
Teacher: OK. But what are antibodies?
Student A: Um. I'm not really sure.
Teacher: Can anyone else tell me?
Student B: Yes, I can. They're substances in the blood that attack things which are foreign to the body, such as the micro-organisms which cause infection.
Teacher: That's it. Yes. And things which cause the body to make antibodies are called antigens, A–N–T–I–G–E–N–S. When the body comes across infective organisms, it produces antibodies against them. This protects it, so that the next time the person comes across the organism, they won't get infected by it.
Student A: But how do you prevent people getting infections in the first place?
Teacher: You can do that by immunising them. There are two types of immunisation, active and passive. Does anyone know what these terms mean?
Student C: Passive means that you inject a person with antibodies against a disease which are taken from someone else. It gives immediate protection.
Teacher: Correct. And what about active immunisation? Perhaps I'd better tell you a bit about it. Active immunisation is also called vaccination. In vaccination, you inject the person with harmless substances which stimulate the body to produce antibodies against a harmful organism. It takes longer to work than passive immunisation, but its effects last a lot longer too. There are three types of vaccination. Firstly, you can use a weakened form of the infective agent. This is what you do with measles and tuberculosis. Secondly, you can use killed organisms. This is what you do with influenza. The third type is for bacteria that cause harm by producing poisons. You inject a safe form of the poison. This is what you do with tetanus T–E–T–A–N–U–S. It's not all that complicated, but it's very important, so you'd better write it down before you forget it. OK?
Student B: Can I ask a question?
Teacher: Yes. What is it?
Student B: What about AIDS? Is there going to be a vaccine against HIV?
Teacher: Well, that's a difficult one to answer. It's possible in theory. Lots of money's being spent on looking for one. So, who knows? There might be a vaccine one day.

KEY

1 ● Immunity is present when the body has formed defences against an infection.
● Antibodies are substances in the blood which attack things foreign to the body, such as micro-organisms
● Antigens are substances which cause the body to make antibodies.
● Passive immunisation is the injection of a person with antibodies against a disease which are taken from someone else.
● Active immunisation involves injecting a person with harmless substances which stimulate the body to produce antibodies against harmful substances or organisms.

2 ● Weakened forms of infective agent, e.g. measles, tuberculosis.
● Killed organisms, e.g. influenza.
● Safe forms of a poison, e.g. tetanus.

3 Passive immunisation takes effect more quickly, but active immunisation affords longer protection.

UNIT 7: PHARMACOLOGY AND THERAPEUTICS

A. Understanding a printed text (1)

KEY

1 Phenylalanine.
2 In the adrenal medulla.
3 Local synthesis and uptake from the extracellular space.
4 Monoamine oxidase (MAO) and catechol-O-methyltransferase (COMT).
5 Stimulus reaction coupling.
6 Stimulate receptors on the presynaptic membrane.

B. Check your understanding

KEY

1 ● incorrect
  ● correct
  ● incorrect
  ● incorrect
  ● correct
  ● incorrect
  ● incorrect
  ● correct
  ● incorrect
  ● correct

2 ● In the cytoplasm of the nerve cell.
  ● Prevention of release of noradrenaline; depletion of noradrenaline stores by prevention of re-uptake; formation of false neurotransmitter; receptor blockade.
  ● Movement across membrane is passive when noradrenaline is passing out of the granules and out of the cell. It is active in the opposite direction.

3 Postsynaptic receptors leading to transmission of the nerve impulse. Presynaptic receptors reducing further transmitter release.

C. Increase your vocabulary

KEY

1 ● enveloped
  ● release
  ● periphery
  ● fuses
  ● ruptures
  ● retained
  ● triggers

2 ● from
  ● on
  ● of
  ● with
  ● by
  ● to
  ● by
  ● from

3 ● limit
  ● regulates
  ● inhibit
  ● influences

D. Check your grammar

KEY

1 from; through; into; to; through; across; on; in; into; through.
2 ● intracellular/extracellular; presynaptic/postsynaptic
  ● insignificant/significant; inactivation/activation
  ● exogenously/endogenously; extraneuronal/intraneuronal; exocytosis/endocytosis
3 ● The shape was asymmetrical.
  ● His inability was obvious.
  ● The point needs to be restated.
  ● Further involvement is undesirable.
  ● Because of war and disease, that area has been depopulated.
  ● The theory has been misapplied.
4 ● Do not take these drugs if you are pregnant.
  ● You should only eat fresh foods.

● If you suffer any strange effects when taking these pills, you should tell your doctor.
● You should never take pills that have not been prescribed by a doctor.
● Keep this bottle out of reach of small children.
● Only telephone your doctor when absolutely necessary.

E. Understanding a lecture

TAPESCRIPT

You will now hear a lecture on factors influencing the action of drugs. As you listen, take notes.

Good afternoon! My lecture today deals with the factors that influence the action of drugs. You might think that once you prescribe a person a pill to swallow, that is the end of the matter. But, in fact, it is much more complicated than that. You have to get the dose right, and you have to alter it according to the patient's response. Some patients need drugs in doses which to others would be poisonous. What, then, are the factors which affect the action of a drug? That is what I shall be talking about today.

▶▶▶

First of all, the patient has actually to take the pills which have been prescribed. This is known as compliance. This might seem an obvious point, but research has shown that millions of pounds worth of drugs prescribed by doctors every year are never in fact taken. I'm sure you've all been prescribed antibiotics at some point. How often have you actually finished the prescribed course? But presuming that the patient has taken the pill, what happens next? Well, this can be influenced by the composition of the tablet itself, known as the formulation. The tablet is not 100% drug. The drug is mixed with other substances and these can influence the rate of absorption of the drug.

▶▶▶

Next comes the process of absorption itself — in other words, the process by which the drug is taken in from the gut into the blood-stream. This can be a passive process or an active process, depending on the chemical structure of the drug. Some drugs, like insulin, cannot be taken by mouth, because they are broken down in the gut before they can be absorbed. Most drugs are absorbed in the upper part of the small bowel, so any disease that interferes with the small bowel will affect absorption of the drug. Once the drug has been absorbed from the gut, the blood in which it is contained has to pass through the liver before it reaches the general circulation. Some drugs are largely destroyed by the liver at this stage, so large doses need to be given. If the liver is diseased, more drug than expected will enter the body.

▶▶▶

Then there is distribution. Once in the body, the drug is distributed around the tissues. Some drugs diffuse freely around the body. Others become attached to proteins. When this happens, it increases the amount of drug that needs to be absorbed before the right concentration in the tissues is reached. Some proteins bind two sorts of drug but prefer one sort to the other. Two drugs may compete for the protein. If the protein is initially bound to the first sort, and then the second sort appears in the blood-stream, the proteins release the first drug. This means that the concentration of the first drug is suddenly increased by taking the second drug. This can be dangerous. As for the protein which binds the drug, it is manufactured in the liver. If the liver is diseased, there will be less of the protein and so smaller doses of the drug will produce higher concentrations of the drug in the blood than would otherwise be the case.

▶▶▶

Finally, we must consider the elimination of the active drug from the body. This happens in two ways; by metabolism and by excretion. Metabolism occurs in the liver, which changes active drugs into inactive substances which can be excreted by the kidney. Some drugs can be excreted directly by the kidney without being metabolised. Any disease that interferes with the liver or the kidney is going to affect the levels of drug achieved by a given dose. And the function of these organs declines with age, so that older people need smaller doses of drugs. And, of course, if a person is taking a drug which interferes with the function of the liver or kidney, this will also affect the elimination of any other drug taken and so affect concentrations in the body and the dosages required. So you see, there is a lot more to it than just swallowing a pill.

KEY
1 ● compliance, formulation, absorption, distribution, elimination

Section 2
● the patient taking the pills as prescribed
● the composition of the tablet

Section 3
● because it is destroyed before it can be absorbed
● more

Section 4
● by diffusion and by binding to proteins

Section 5
● metabolism and excretion
● they should be reduced
2 ● poisonous
● from the gut into the blood-stream
● the upper part of the small bowel
● the liver
● the liver
● inactive substances; the kidney
3 *Small bowel* — prevents absorption so reducing blood concentration.
Liver — decreased metabolism allows more drug to reach the circulation and slows rate of elimination thereby increasing drug concentration.
— reduced production of carrier proteins, thereby increasing the concentration of the free fraction of drugs usually bound to proteins.
Kidney — reduced excretion may lead to higher blood concentrations.
4 No key is possible.

G. Check your understanding

KEY
1 ● having a healthy effect on mind and body
● looking back at past events
● deadly
● recovering from illness
● too ready to believe things
● a patented name, e.g. 'Contergan' for thalidomide
● causing congenital malformity

2 ● because thalidomide was marketed in West Germany for two years longer than in Britain
● five years and three years respectively
● hands and feet come straight from the body with virtually no arms or legs
● they thought the drug was too obviously innocent to be worth mentioning
● it was safe in overdose
● because it was sold mixed with other drugs in simple household remedies with proprietary names.
3 Drugs can have serious and unexpected side-effects and these can take years to become apparent.
4 No key is possible.

H. Understanding discourse

TAPESCRIPT
Listen to somebody reading the instructions on a monoamine-oxidase inhibitor treatment card.

TREATMENT CARD
Carry this card with you at all times. Show it to any doctor who may treat you other than the doctor who prescribed this medicine, and to your dentist if you require dental treatment.

INSTRUCTIONS TO PATIENTS
Please read carefully
While taking this medicine and for 14 days after your treatment finishes you must observe the following simple instructions:-

1 Do not eat CHEESE, PICKLED HERRING OR BROAD BEAN PODS.
2 Do not eat or drink BOVRIL, OXO, MARMITE or ANY SIMILAR MEAT OR YEAST EXTRACT.
3 Eat only FRESH foods and avoid food that you suspect could be stale or 'going off'. This is especially important with meat, fish, poultry or offal. Avoid game.
4 Do not take any other MEDICINES (including tablets, capsules, nose drops, inhalations or suppositories) whether purchased by you or previously prescribed by your doctor, without first consulting your doctor or your pharmacist.

NB *Treatment for coughs and colds, pain relievers, tonics and laxatives are medicines.*
5 Avoid alcoholic drinks.

Keep a careful note of any food or drink that disagrees with you, avoid it and tell your doctor.

Report any unusual or severe symptoms to your doctor and follow any other advice given by him.

KEY
1 Carry it with you at all times. Show it to any new doctor or to your dentist.
2 While taking the medicine and for 14 days after treatment finishes.
3 Certain foods; alcoholic drink; medicines.
4 *Nota bene* (Latin) = note carefully.
5 Report them to your doctor.
6 *You must observe* the following simple instructions.

A. Understanding a printed text (1)

KEY

1 History, physical examination, special examinations, diagnosis, treatment.
2 Adenoma sebaceum.
3 Subungual fibroma.
4 Adenoma sebaceum, epilepsy and mental deficiency.
5 No.

B. Check your understanding

KEY

1 She did very badly at school.
2 Because the mother was embarrassed by the eruption.
3 Three or four years.
4 The occurrence of a nocturnal seizure.
5 No.
6 Psychometric testing; skull radiographs; computerised tomography of the head.
7 Epiloia.
8 Yes.
9 For control of epilepsy.
10 In institutional care.

C. Increase your vocabulary

KEY

1 revealed, showed, disclosed, furnished
2 ● parietal bones/skull
  ● subungual fibromas/fingers
  ● phakoma of the retina/eye
  ● renal lesions/kidney
  ● lateral ventricles/brain
  ● shagreen patches/back
  ● distal phalanges/hands or feet
  ● cheeks/face
3 1h, 2k, 3a, 4l, 5b, 6j, 7m, 8c, 9d, 10i, 11e, 12g, 13f

D. Check your grammar

KEY

1 Sample answers
  ● Both fresh vegetables and fried food are common constituents in the European diet. Compared with fried food, fresh vegetables are much heathier.
  ● Water and ice are both forms of the same substance. Ice is more rigid in structure compared with water.
  ● Neither alcohol nor heroin are good for one's health. In comparison with heroin, alcohol is far more readily available in most parts of the world.
  ● Both measles and AIDS are caused by viral infections. Compared with AIDS, measles is a mild disease.
  ● Neither aspirin nor thalidomide were difficult to obtain in the late 1950s. Compared with thalidomide, aspirin is a safe drug in normal dosages.
2 Sample answers
  ● Overnutrition is common in Europe, while undernutrition is common in parts of Africa.

● Diarrhoeal diseases are not widespread in developed countries. However, they are common in underdeveloped countries.
● Carbohydrate is composed of sugar molecules. Protein, on the other hand, is made up of amino acids.
● Helminths are worms, whereas protozoa are unicellular organisms.
3 ● Helminths, that is worms, are commoner in countries with poor sanitation, lack of clean water and so on, leading to more parasitic disease and chronic infestation. Therefore, improvements in public health (see below), including treatment with drugs, for example piperazine, are necessary to control the problem.
  ● Anti-convulsants e.g. phenytoin now used in treatment of epilepsy i.e. recurrent fits → great improvement in life-style & general health ∴ prognosis for those c̄ epilepsy usually good.
  ● See text.

E. Understanding a lecture

TAPESCRIPT

Good morning! There are three main elements in the gathering of information upon which to form a diagnosis. These are: the history, the physical examination and special investigations. Each is approached in a logical order, which remains much the same every time that the process is gone through. History-taking begins with the patient giving his own account of the problem in his own words. The doctor will then seek clarification about particular details, such as the exact character and duration of the symptoms. There follows questioning about the patient's past, in particular his previous illnesses and the presence or absence of disease in his family. Details are then taken of his personal life and social circumstances and of the drugs he is taking, both social and medicinal. At the end, the doctor usually goes through a check-list of symptoms relating to the different organ systems of the body — respiratory, cardiovascular, genito-urinary, gastro-intestinal, neurological and so on. By this stage, the doctor should have enough information to decide which diagnoses are likely.

▶▶▶

The physical examination is used to confirm and refine the diagnosis. It is conducted in a standardised fashion, beginning with the general appearance of the patient and then going through each system in turn. More time may be spent on areas in which abnormalities are expected and less on areas likely to remain unaffected, but no area must be left unexplored or important information may be missed. By the end of the examination, the doctor will have discovered a pattern of abnormalities, which indicate a specific diagnosis.

▶▶▶

Sometimes it is necessary to obtain further information to assist in diagnosis and treatment, by the use of special investigations. The range of these is wide, and the doctor in a large hospital may be able to call upon the services of a small army of experts and technicians. Let's look at a list of a few of these investigative methods on this overhead slide. The list is really self-explanatory. Haematology involves the study of the constituents of the blood. Biochemistry involves examination of various chemicals in the blood or other body fluids which reflect the state of body organs, such as the liver and kidneys. Microbiology laboratories examine and culture micro-organisms from samples taken from patients. Histologists examine tissue samples from patients.

There is a wide range of radiological techniques which allow imaging of the interior of the body. I expect you are familiar with most of these terms. Contrast studies involve the injection of radio-opaque liquid into the body to outline structures; an example is angiography, in which the course of blood vessels is examined. Nuclear imaging involves the use of radioactively labelled substances to delineate organs such as the lungs and brain. Then there are the highly specialised techniques. Computerised axial tomography known as CT scanning is available in large hospitals. The remaining techniques, NMR and PET scanning, remain prohibitively expensive and are used mainly as tools in specialised research. Lastly, we should mention special instrumental techniques, such as gastroscopy in which the stomach is visualised through a flexible fibreoptic tube passed down the oesophagus. Similar instruments are used for examining the interior of other bodily orifices.

KEY

1 ● history, physical examination and special investigations
  ● the patient's account of the problem; clarification of details by the doctor; previous illnesses; disease in the family; personal life; social circumstances; drugs; check-list of symptoms
  ● after taking a history
  ● to confirm and refine the diagnosis
  ● the general appearance of the patient
  ● the ones in which abnormalities are expected
  ● important information may otherwise be missed
  ● they are prohibitively expensive
2 *haematology* — the study of the constituents of the blood
  biochemistry — examination of chemicals in the blood or other body fluids.
  microbiology — examination and culture of micro-organisms from patient samples
  histology — the examination of tissue samples from patients
  radiology — imaging the interior of the body
  contrast techniques — the injection of radio-opaque liquids into the body to outline structures
  nuclear imaging — the use of radioactively labelled substances to delineate organs
  gastroscopy — visualisation of the stomach through a flexible fibreoptic tube passed down the oesophagus

G. Check your understanding

KEY

1 ● incorrect
  ● incorrect
  ● incorrect
  ● correct
  ● incorrect
  ● incorrect
  ● correct
  ● incorrect
  ● correct
  ● incorrect
  ● correct
  ● correct
2 ● the central nervous system
  ● no
  ● disuse
  ● partial or complete loss of vision coming on over a period of hours or days; sometimes pain in the eye
  ● steroids
  ● as sunflower seed oil

H. Understanding discourse

Listen to this conversation. Dr Etherington, a junior doctor, is in the middle of a ward round with his consultant.

Consultant: Are you asleep? Come on! Wake up!

Dr Etherington: What? Oh. Right. Sorry. I've been up for 72 hours so far. Only another 8 hours to work and I'll be able to go to bed.

Consultant: Being a houseman's not that bad. We had to go through it all, as well, you know. Good for the soul. Anyway, who's the new man in bed seventeen?

Dr Etherington: That's Charles Spence, a 56-year-old married chartered accountant from Wimbledon. He presented to casualty on Friday night having had three car accidents in the last three days. On each occasion, the other car was coming from the left and he says he simply didn't see them coming. All the accidents occurred in daylight and he doesn't drink.

Consultant: What did you find on examination?

Dr Etherington: He's got no remaining vision in the left half of his visual field. There's some sensory loss in the right arm, but no other neurological abnormalities.

Consultant: What do you think the problem is?

Dr Etherington: He appears to have a lesion in his left occipital cortex which is beginning to extend into the parietal region. Since he hasn't any history of vascular disease, I suspect he has a brain tumour.

Consultant: Yes. It sounds like it. Have you booked a CT scan?

Dr Etherington: Yes. He's having one this afternoon.

Consultant: Right. Let's have a quick word with him . . . Hello, Mr Spence. Dr Etherington has just been telling me all about you. Nothing to worry about. We'll soon have you back at work. Good-bye for now . . . He'll be dead in three months, wouldn't you say, Dr Etherington?

Dr Etherington: I'm afraid you're probably right.

Consultant: If the scan shows tumour, you'd better start him on some steroids. Book a bed in the neurosurgical ward for a brain biopsy. And you'd better have a word with his wife before you go off duty. If you need me I'll be in Harley Street. Cheerio.

KEY

1 Because he has been working for 72 hours without sleep.
2 He suffered three car accidents in three days.
3 No remaining vision in his left visual field; some sensory loss in the right arm.
4 Tumour.
5 Vascular disease.
6 A CT scan.
7 It is not true.
8 Steroids and a brain biopsy.

UNIT 9: PSYCHIATRY

A. Understanding a printed text (1)

KEY

1 A subjective sense of well-being accompanied by increased activity.
2 Irritability.
3 Flight of ideas.
4 A lowering of mood accompanied by a reduction in energy and activity.
5 Anhedonia.
6 Retardation.

B. Check your understanding

KEY

1 No exact key is possible. A suggested table is as follows:

	Mania	Melancholia
Mood	Subjective sense of wellbeing Elated and/or irritable or uncharacteristic equanimity Depression beneath surface	Lowering of mood Gloomy Diurnal variation Sad. Unhappy
Energy	Abundant	Reduced energy and activity
Effectiveness	Achieves little, too distractible Impaired judgement	Poor
Sleep	Stays up late, rises early Not tired	Early morning wakening Tired
Behaviour	Poor judgement. Squanders large sums of money. Uninhibited, especially sexual behaviour	Anhedonia. Abandons normal recreations. Libido and appetite decreased Retarded movements
Thought	Can think more clearly than ever before. Head full of plans and ideas. Grandiose ideas or delusions	Restricted to a few gloomy themes
Speech	Pressure of speech	Retarded. Restricted in quantity and limited in range. Quiet, dull monotonous voice.
Delusions	Grandiose in nature	Guilty in nature
Suicide risk	By no means rare	Ever present
View of future	Wonderful	No future
Other symptoms		Loss of weight Agitation common Poor concentration and attention Hallucinations may occur

2 No key is possible. It is advisable to check the tables constructed by the students before they engage upon this exercise. It could be used as a class exercise rather than a written exercise if this is thought desirable.
3 Upper pair: depression. Lower pair: mania. No further key is possible. The description should be regarded as an exercise in the use of adjectives and abstracts and in exact choice of language.

C. Increase your vocabulary

KEY

1 sadness, depression, gloom, guilt, elation, irritability
2 ● 1h, 2f, 3b, 4j, 5c, 6d, 7e, 8g, 9a, 10i

D. Check your grammar

KEY

1 ● severity, awareness, confidence
● gloomy, melancholic
● obviously, casually
● desirable, embarrassing
● interaction, impairment, agitation
2 ● Such patients are often preoccupied with minor indiscretions from the past.
● Manics are frequently distractible.
● When a patient fails to be alarmed by bad news, this may indicate that his mood is elevated.

E. Understanding a lecture

TAPESCRIPT

You are going to hear a lecture about how to perform a psychiatric examination.

Good afternoon, ladies and gentlemen! How do you examine a patient to look for psychiatric illness? Well, in many ways, it's similar to examining a patient with a physical illness. You still find out what the patient is complaining of before you examine them, and when examining them you go through the parts to be examined in a logical order. What you're examining is the person's state of mind at the time that you see them. This is known as the mental state. But, in one way, examination of the mental state is obviously very different from examination of the body. You are dealing with things that have no physical form. In other words, they are abstract. There are no lumps or bumps to feel or prod. You can't look into the mind with any instrument. You simply have to use your powers of observation and your skill in analysing what people say.

▶▶▶

The mental state examination falls into a number of parts, and we'll go through these one by one. You begin by examining the person's appearance and behaviour. This means what they look like and what they do at interview. They may be dressed in a peculiar way, or react to the situation in a way which is quite inappropriate. You then consider their speech. They may not speak at all, or they may speak terribly fast or use words that don't exist. Next comes their thought. First, you look at the form of their thought. Can you follow it? Some people may jump from idea to idea in a way that doesn't make sense. For instance, in mania, they may switch from one subject to another simply because two words rhyme. It may be quite impossible to understand what they're talking about. The patient himself may have funny ideas about his thoughts. He may think they belong to someone else, or that everyone else can read them or that they're being broadcast on radio or TV. Such ideas generally indicate a diagnosis of schizophrenia. After considering the form of thought, you can look at the content of a person's thought. Does he have any strange ideas or beliefs that are evidently not true? Some people might believe, for example, that their movements are being followed by small green men from the planet Mars. Such a false belief is called a delusion.

▶▶▶

Next you go on to look at their perceptions. That means what they are told by their senses — hearing, seeing, smelling and so on. Some people hear voices when there is no one there. This can be very upsetting. And some people feel compelled to do what the voices tell them. Perceptions in the absence of any form of stimulus are known as hallucinations. Hallucinations of hearing are called auditory hallucinations. You can get hallucinations of any modality of sensation — seeing visions, smelling strange odours and so on.

▶▶▶

There are three more areas of a person's mental function that you look at. Firstly, their mood. Are they depressed, anxious or elated? Then you look at their cognitive state. This means their mental processes, such as memory and concentration. Some people, for instance, might be able to remember very little. They might not know where they are or what day it is. Such abnormalities often indicate a physical disease which is affecting the brain. Lastly, you look at their insight. This means their ability to see their situation for what it is. Many people who have delusions or hallucinations do not believe they are ill. In other words, they lack insight.

▶▶▶

At the end of your examination, you probably have a list of abnormalities. You then fit these together in a pattern and look for the illness that this pattern fits best. This gives you the diagnosis. Sometimes it's easy and sometimes it's difficult. The only way to learn it is by watching someone else do it, and then practising it yourself.

KEY
1 *Section 1*—————————————————————
  ● You find out what the patient is complaining of before you examine them, and when examining them you go through the parts to be examined in a logical order.
  ● You are dealing with abstracts rather than lumps or bumps.
  ● the mental state examination
  Section 2—————————————————————
  ● mania
  ● schizophrenia
  ● a delusion
  Section 3—————————————————————
  ● what a person is told by their senses
  ● an hallucination
  Section 4—————————————————————
  ● physical disease
  ● the ability to see the situation for what it is
2 Appearance and behaviour; speech; thought — form of thought and content of thought; perceptions; mood; cognitive state; insight.
  For definitions, no exact key is possible.

G. Check your understanding

KEY
1 ● that the girl has very affectionate feelings towards the student
  ● because it would have been very embarrassing for the girl and far more than she would have wished anyone to know at the time
  ● from subsequent events
  ● worry about difficulties in his life
  ● It is an apparently irrelevant incident that shows an obvious parallel to another situation which is highly relevant, and of which the person might well be wanting to speak, without being aware of it.
2 No key is possible
3 messsage/message (paragraph 3, line 6)

H. Understanding discourse

TAPESCRIPT
Fred and Joe are discussing a lecture that they have just attended on the classification of psychiatric disorder.

Fred: Hello Joe. How did you enjoy that lecture?
Joe: I enjoyed it alright, but I got a bit lost towards the end.
Fred: Where was that, then?
Joe: In the last few minutes, when he was talking about the classification of psychiatric illness. The lecturer was speaking so fast that I couldn't get it all written down.
Fred: I think I managed to get it all down. Here. Have a look at my notes.
Joe: Thanks. Now, where are we?
Fred: I think the part you want starts here, on side seven.
Joe: Oh, yes. That's it. Where he's talking about psychosis and neurosis. That was difficult. I think I understand neurosis. That's where people have feelings we all experience, like anxiety or depression, but they have them more severely or more often than they ought to. Is that right?
Fred: Yes, that's more or less it. What about psychosis?
Joe: Ah, well that's where I got lost. Can you explain it?
Fred: Sure. People with psychoses are the really crazy ones. They have bizarre experiences that most people never have. Hallucinations, delusions and that sort of thing.
Joe: OK. What about this diagram, though? I didn't manage to get it all filled in.
Fred: Well, if you take the psychoses, there are two main types, organic and functional. Organic means that the illness is due to a physical disease, such as infection or drug intoxication. I'm not so sure what functional means.
Joe: Perhaps it just means that no-one can find the cause, though presumably there must be one.
Fred: Yeah, I think you're right.
Joe: And what are the two types of functional psychosis?
Fred: Er. There's affective disorder — that means to do with the mood. Then there's schizophrenia. But look at the affective ones again. They're split into two types, mania and depression.
Joe: OK. But why have I put that two-way arrow on the diagram?
Fred: That's just to show that some people get episodes of both mania and depression at different times.
Joe: Great. Thanks. I think that's all I missed. I've had quite enough psychiatry for one morning. I'll buy you a cup of coffee.
Fred: Thanks. Good idea.

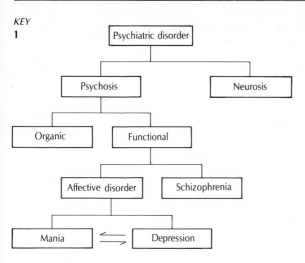

2 In psychosis, people have bizarre experiences such as hallucinations and delusions which most people never experience. In neurosis, people have feelings that everyone experiences, such as anxiety or depression, but they have them more severely or more often than they ought to.

3 Organic psychoses are the result of an identifiable physical disease. In functional psychoses, no physical pathology is evident.

UNIT 10: PAEDIATRICS

A. Understanding a printed text (1)

KEY
1 1 in 2000
2 It is inherited as an autosomal recessive condition.
3 Meconium ileus, recurrent lung infections, malabsorption.
4 A form of neonatal small bowel obstruction, due to thick viscid meconium.
5 Postural drainage.

B. Check your understanding

KEY
1 1. Chronic suppurative lung disease.
   2. 1 in 25
   3. A defect in ciliary mechanism.
   4. In infancy.
   5. By finding increased sodium and chloride levels in sweat obtained by pilocarpine iontophoresis.
   6. Surgical treatment.
   7. Overdistension of the lungs and peribronchial thickening.
   8. *Pseudomonas* and *Staphylococcus aureus*.
   9. By giving pancreatic enzyme supplements with meals.
   10. Cirrhosis and diabetes.
   11. 1 in 4
   12. 60–65%
2 No key is possible.

C. Increase your vocabulary

KEY
1 ● commonest
   ● infertility
   ● obstruction
   ● recurrent
2 ● diagnosis before birth
   ● testing all the newborn to find those few with a particular problem

● giving advice to prospective parents about their risks of producing children with inherited abnormalities
3 1h, 2e, 3f, 4a, 5c, 6k, 7j, 8d, 9b, 10g, 11i

D. Check your grammar

KEY
1 have made
2 had
3 has been better understood
4 improved
5 was elucidated
6 have been
7 have not yet been developed
8 was once thought

E. Understanding a lecture

TAPESCRIPT

You will now hear part of a lecture on the subject of acute stridor.

Good afternoon! The subject of today's lecture is acute stridor. Acute, in this context, means of sudden onset. Stridor is one of the most important signs of respiratory illness in children. It is a harsh sound caused by obstruction at the level of the upper airway — that is to say the larynx or trachea. The important thing to remember is that it is an inspiratory noise. Here it differs from that other important respiratory noise, the wheeze. Remember that a wheeze is a softer sound, occurring on expiration, and originating from obstruction of the lower airways, known as bronchioles. Stridor is an important subject to consider because there are several different causes which range from the relatively benign to the life-threatening.

▶▶▶

So let's just run through a short list of causes, before considering the main ones in detail. The first to consider is croup or acute laryngo-tracheo-bronchitis, which is by far the most common. Rarer, but important, causes are acute epiglottitis and the inhalation of a foreign body. Rarer still are some more obscure conditions such as angioneurotic oedema, an allergic condition causing swelling of the face and larynx. Diphtheria was once a common cause, but is now rare since the introduction of immunisation in infancy.

▶▶▶

Croup as its longer name suggests is an inflammation of the larynx, trachea and bronchi. It is caused by a viral infection, which leads to the narrowing of the airway due to mucosal oedema and secretions. Typically, the child is between the ages of 1 and 3 years. He has had a cold for a few days and the mother has noticed a 'croupy' cough which is worse at night or when the child cries. Otherwise, the child is usually not very unwell and only has a mild temperature. Sometimes the attack may be more severe. This is indicated by the severity of the stridor, by an increase in heart rate and respiratory rate and by the degree of intercostal recession — that is to say, how hard the child is having to breathe in order to overcome the upper airway obstruction. In severe attacks or when the child is exhausted, then he should be admitted to hospital for observation. Otherwise, if the parents are confident, then the child can be cared for at home and the parents instructed to watch for signs of deterioration. Of those children admitted to hospital, one per cent need intubation — in other words, the insertion of a tube into the trachea to stop it blocking.

▶▶▶

In a small but important group of children, the pattern of stridor is different. The stridor is more severe and it is associated with a high temperature. Typically, the child is between the ages of 3 to 7 years, is very unwell and is sitting forwards drooling because he cannot swallow. The condition is called acute epiglottitis and is caused by infection of the epiglottis with the bacterium, *Haemophilus influenzae*. This is an extremely dangerous condition, and, if it is suspected, admission to hospital is mandatory. Some paediatricians intubate all such children for 24 hours, because there is a real danger of the swollen epiglottis completely blocking the child's airway. In fact, the cardinal rule in examining any child with stridor is *never* to examine the throat as this may cause the airway to obstruct. Treatment of acute epiglottitis is with intravenous antibiotics.

▶▶▶

Last but not least comes inhalation of a foreign body. Toddlers are curious by nature, and enjoy putting objects like safety pins and buttons into their mouths. The diagnosis is usually revealed by a careful history. Often there has been a short fit of coughing when a child has been playing with small objects. Peanuts are well-known culprits. There is no temperature and the child, unless seriously obstructed, is not unwell. Sometimes the presence of a foreign body can be revealed on X-ray, but some objects such as peanuts are radiolucent. It is often necessary to proceed to laryngoscopy, in which a surgeon passes a small fibre-optic instrument into the airway to visualise the object directly. It can then be removed with special instruments.

KEY
Section 1————————————————————————
● Stridor is a harsh inspiratory sound produced by narrowing of the upper airway, whereas wheeze is a softer expiratory sound, originating from obstruction of the lower airways.

Section 2————————————————————————
● croup or acute laryngo-tracheo-bronchitis; acute epiglottitis; inhalation of a foreign body; angioneurotic oedema; diphtheria

Section 3————————————————————————
● mucosal oedema and secretions
● severe stridor, increased heart and respiratory rates, intercostal recession

● in severe attacks or when exhausted
● one per cent

Section 4————————————————————————
● admission to hospital
● never examine the throat

Section 5————————————————————————
● by taking a careful history
● because peanuts are radiolucent

	Croup	Acute epiglottitis	Inhalation of a foreign body
Age	1–3	3–7	Toddler
Typical presentation	A cold for a few days with a croupy cough	Sitting forward drooling, unable to swallow	Recent fit of coughing when playing with small objects
Temperature	Mild	Severe	None
Causative agent	Virus	*Haemophilus influenzae*	Foreign body
Part of respiratory tract affected	Trachea, larynx, bronchi	Epiglottis	Varies
Management	Observation	Hospitalisation Intravenous antibiotics Sometimes intubation	Removal of object

G. Check your understanding

KEY
1 ● incorrect   ● correct
   ● correct   ● incorrect
   ● incorrect   ● incorrect
   ● incorrect   ● correct
   ● incorrect   ● incorrect
2 upper respiratory tract infections; prolonged exercise; inhaled allergens; emotional factors; changes in the weather
3 subcutaneous, intramuscular, intravenous

H. Understanding discourse

TAPESCRIPT
You are going to hear the discussion at a case conference in the paediatric department of the hospital. Listen carefully to what is said.

Chairman: OK, everyone. Let's get started. I'd better begin by introducing myself. I'm Damian from the hospital social services department and I'm chairing this case conference today because Barbara, who was chairman last time, is off sick. I presume you all know each other, as you were all present at the first case confrence two months ago. Trevor, perhaps you'd like to start by reminding us what we're here for.

Trevor: Right, as you know, I'm the social worker attached to the paediatric department. The purpose of our meeting today is to discuss what to do about Ashley Smith, aged ten, who for the last year has refused to attend school. He has spent the days at home with his mother and two-year-old baby sister. The situation is complicated by his asthma, which has been very bad over the last year. Is that not so, Dr Angel?

Dr Angel: Indeed, Ashley's been admitted four times in the last year dangerously ill. He has spent a total of two months in hospital and he needs careful looking after.

Chairman: Does that in itself mean that it's physically difficult for him to take part in normal school activities?

Dr Angel: No, not as such. He needs to use his two inhalers four times a day, and it might not be a good idea for him to take part in sports. But between episodes, his physical state is quite good. I think the problem's a psychological one really. He's very anxious when separated from his mother — partly because he hated being in hospital so much and partly because he's terrified of the illness itself.

Trevor: What about the mother? Rebecca, you're the family aide and visit them regularly. Have you anything you want to tell us?

Rebecca: Yes. The problem is that the mother's single and that Archibald, Ashley's elder brother, died from a severe asthmatic attack two years ago. I think the mother's afraid of losing Ashley too and she colludes with his staying off school.

Dr Angel: Yes, and another problem is that Ashley's asthma is made worse by stress; and if we force him to go to school, it will make his asthma worse.

Chairman: What do you think we should do then?

Dr Angel: Well, normally I would recommend a gradual return to school — perhaps starting for a few hours at a time. But in this instance, we have to be a bit more careful, because we need to get the mother's co-operation before we can hope to have any success. It was a pity that she wasn't invited to this meeting. I think Rebecca and I should talk to her together and report back on progress in six weeks' time.

Chairman: Alright. Everyone agreed on that? Good. We'll reconvene in six weeks at the same time in the same room. See you all then.

KEY

1 chairman of the case conference
2 by introducing himself
3 yes, one
4 she is ill
5 to discuss what to do about Ashley Smith, aged ten, who for the last year has refused to attend school
6 two years old
7 two months
8 two weeks
9 two inhalers four times a day
10 he is anxious about leaving his mother
11 because she has already lost one child due to severe asthma
12 his asthma might get worse
13 sports
14 that Dr Angel and Rebecca will talk to the mother, then report back to a further meeting in six weeks' time
15 Damian — chairman
   Trevor — social worker
   Dr Angel — doctor
   Rebecca — family aide
16 OK, right, well, alright

CHECK YOUR PROGRESS (2)

A. Reading

KEY
The following answers are correct:

1 a. c.	5 a.
2 a. e.	6 b. d. e.
3 a. c. e.	7 c. d. e.
4 a. b. d.	8 d. e.

B. Writing

KEY
It may be useful to remind students of different ways of expressing descriptive information, for instance, by providing alternatives to the verb 'to be'. Similarly, for the comparison of two types of pain, the students might be reminded of connecting words, such as *whereas, however, in contrast to, unlike,* etc.

C. Listening

TAPESCRIPT
You will now hear part of a lecture about heart failure. It is divided into four sections.

Heart failure is the condition that results when the efficiency of the heart as a pump is decreased. There are two sorts of heart failure, right heart failure and left heart failure. This is because the heart really consists of two pumps. The right heart receives blood from the body and pumps it through the lungs, where carbon dioxide is released and oxygen absorbed. The left heart receives blood from the lungs and pumps it round the body. The left part of the heart is stronger than the right.

The symptoms and signs of heart failure are generally distant from the heart itself. Right heart failure produces different symptoms to left heart failure, although the two may occur together. The symptoms in heart failure are caused by back pressure from the heart which is not clearing blood quickly enough. In right heart failure, there is increased pressure in the veins returning blood to the heart. This can be seen in the jugular vein in the neck, which should be examined with the patient propped up at an angle of 30°. In right heart failure, the vein is distended with blood. In the absence of failure, it is not. Back pressure from the right heart has many other effects. Fluid is squeezed into the tissues of the legs and into the abdomen, which swell with fluid. This swelling is known as oedema. The liver becomes swollen with blood and enlarged in size. This enlargement can be felt when examining the patient's abdomen, and the liver is often found to be tender. The patient may have little appetite because of congestion in the veins of the gut, and weight loss often occurs. The kidneys become less efficient as a result of increased venous pressure, and urine output drops.

In left heart failure, the back pressure results in congestion of the lungs. Here, also, oedema results. Fluid in the lungs produces audible sounds which can be found on listening to the chest with a stethoscope. Oedema causes breathlessness which may come on suddenly and be extremely frightening to the sufferer. The breathlessness is characteristically worse when lying flat, a phenomenon known as orthopnoea. Patients with chronic left heart failure often describe having to sleep propped up in bed with lots of pillows. The back pressure from the failing left heart increases the amount of work that has to be done by the right heart to pump blood through the lungs. In this way, left heart failure may result in right heart failure.

▶▶▶

There are many causes of heart failure. These can be divided into three groups, according to the mechanism by which heart failure is produced. The first is an increase in after-load. This means an increase in the pressure necessary to eject blood from the heart. It occurs in high blood pressure or hypertension. It also occurs if the valves at the exit of the heart have become narrowed. Secondly, there is disease of the heart muscle itself which decreases its strength and efficiency. This is most commonly produced by ischaemic heart disease, when the coronary arteries supplying the heart become narrowed. The third mechanism that produces failure is excessive pre-load. This means that the heart has more blood

than usual to pump. This can occur when the heart valves become incompetent and blood which has already been pumped leaks back into the heart. It also occurs in diseases in which the blood must be pumped through the system faster such as beri-beri, chronic anaemia and thyrotoxicosis.

KEY
Section 1
● right and left
● receives blood from the body and pumps it through the lungs
● receives blood from the lungs and pumps it round the body
● the left heart

Section 2
● back pressure
● a. c.

Section 3
● b. c. f.

Section 4
The answers are evident in the above text.

UNIT 11: ONCOLOGY

A. Understanding a printed text (1)

KEY
1 Carcinomas, which are malignant neoplasms of epithelial linings of organs such as the gut and the bronchi.
2 Inheritance and environment.
3 Scotland, England and Wales.
4 By biopsy of the tumour.
5 More than 50% reduction in the size of the tumour.

B. Check your understanding

KEY
1   1. Cardiovascular disease.
   2. Children.
   3. Aflatoxin is a toxic material formed by a mould on groundnuts. It causes liver cancer (hepatoma).
   4. T cell leukaemias; geographical clustering gave the vital clue.
   5. Chimney sweeps.
   6. As one abnormal cell.
   7. A subjective response is one perceived by the sufferer, whereas an objective response is one that the observer makes and is usually associated with some form of measurement.
   8. As the clinical disappearance of all evidence of malignancy with no evidence of tumour presence using the appropriate investigations.
2 Sample answer:
   The figure shows changing incidences of cancers of the stomach and lung and of leukaemia in the male population over the years 1930 to 1965. During this period, the incidence of stomach cancer declined from 30 to 10 per 100,000 male population. The incidence of lung cancer increased from 3 to 35 per 100,000. The incidence of leukaemia increased from 3 to 7 per 100,000.

C. Increase your vocabulary

KEY
1 Variation, proof, induction, remission, response
2 Angiogenesis; hepatoma, mesothelioma
3 Median: the middle number in a series of numbers
   Mean: the average of a series of numbers
4 1d, 2a, 3e, 4c, 5b
5 Response indicates some degree of improvement as a result of treatment.
   Remission means that the disease is in full retreat, but may not have been permanently conquered.
   Cure is the permanent eradication of the disease.

D. Check your grammar

KEY
1 No key is possible.
2 No key is possible.
3 ● If I had been there, I would have done it differently.
   ● If I could, I would play tennis every day.
   ● He could have studied medicine, if he hadn't decided to go abroad instead.
   ● They should have explained everything in detail, if they wanted us to understand.
   ● If you want to buy an expensive dress, you should make sure that you have enough money in the bank first.

E. Understanding a lecture

TAPESCRIPT
You will now hear a lecture on the treatment of cancer.

Good afternoon! Now, we've already looked at some general aspects of cancers. In this lecture, we'll go on to consider the principles of treatment. We can look at this under two headings — local treatment and systemic treatment. Systemic means involving the whole body. Both sorts of treatment are necessary in most cases. The cancer begins and grows in one particular site but it isn't enough simply to treat that site. This is because the tumour sheds cells into the blood stream and lymphatic system. These travel to other locations in the body and begin to grow there. Unless all these cancerous cells are killed, there will be no possibility of cure.

▶▶▶

The main local form of treatment is surgery. The surgeon operates on the patient and tries to cut out as much of the tumour as possible. Sometimes, all visible tumour can be cut out or resected. In other cases, the tumour may have invaded nearby structures in the body and so cannot be fully removed without extensive and mutilating surgery. Nevertheless, it is important to remove as much as possible so as to increase the chances of killing off the tumour by other methods. Sometimes specialised surgical techniques are used such as laser surgery in which the tissue is literally burnt away. Lasers have the advantage of great accuracy and of sealing small blood vessels.

▶▶▶

The second local form of treatment is radiation therapy or radiotherapy. Beams of high voltage radiation are directed at the area of the tumour. The problem is to kill the cancerous cells without damaging the normal healthy tissues of the body. This can be partly achieved by directing several lower-dose beams of radiation at a tumour from different angles. In this way, normal tissues receive only small doses, while the tumour where the beams cross receives higher doses. But not all tumours are sensitive to the effects of radiation, and so it is far less effective in some sorts of cancer than in others. Sometimes, radiotherapy and surgery are used together in the treatment of a localised tumour, because the two together can be more effective than one alone.

▶▶▶

But even if a tumour has been completely ressected or has shrunk away with radiotherapy, it's still likely that some tumour cells will have travelled elsewhere in the body, where they'll have seeded and be silently growing. For this reason, the last twenty years have seen a great expansion in cancer chemotherapy, which means treatment with drugs. These drugs are known as cytotoxic drugs, because they kill cells. They work by killing the tumour cells when they are dividing. But they also kill other dividing cells and so are very poisonous. They suppress the bone marrow, thus interfering with the formation of blood components and with resistance to infection. They make the patient feel extremely ill with nausea and vomiting and diarrhoea, and all the patient's hair falls out. Also, tumours can quickly develop resistance to one drug used alone, so several drugs are usually used in combination. So far, cancer chemotherapy has not been particularly successful. In a few sorts of cancer, chemotherapy can produce a total cure. But in most cancers, the effects are limited and the eventual progression of the disease is not stopped. In the least favourable cases, the misery caused to the patient by the drugs is probably not worth the very short time by which death is postponed.

▶▶▶

But let's turn to something more optimistic. The most exciting developments in cancer therapy have to do with the immune system and with genetic engineering. This is usually known as biological therapy. There have been attempts for many years to find ways of stimulating the body's own defences to attack cancer cells. Recent research has concentrated on techniques of producing antibodies against cancers in the laboratory, the so-called monoclonal antibodies. There is a possibility that these can be

injected into a patient to attack a tumour directly. Also, drugs could be attached to the antibodies. The drugs would then be delivered only to the cancer cells. The problems of poisoning normal cells could be avoided and much higher doses achieved in the tumour itself. It is this technique that offers the most promise for the future.

KEY

1 *Section 1*
- Because the tumour sheds cells into the blood stream which then begin to grow in other parts of the body
Section 2
- Because it may have invaded nearby body structures
- Great accuracy; sealing of small blood vessels
Section 3
- By using several beams of lower dose radiation which cross at the point of the tumour
Section 4
- By killing cells when they are dividing.
- They suppress the bone marrow, interfering with the formation of blood components and with resistance to infection; nausea, vomiting, diarrhoea; hair loss.
- Because tumours quickly develop resistance to one drug used alone.
Section 5
- Because the drugs would be delivered only to the cancer cells and poisoning of normal cells would be avoided.

2 Methods of cancer treatment
  Local
  - surgery
  - radiotherapy
  Systemic
  - chemotherapy
  - biological therapy

3 No key is possible. This is a common dilemma for cancer patients and their relatives. This question could be used as a written exercise or as a subject for class discussion.

G. Check your understanding

KEY

1 1. 1 in 180,000
   2. In acute leukaemias, blast cells are present in the peripheral blood, whereas in chronic leukaemias excessive numbers of normal-looking leucocytes are present.
   3. Those with Down's syndrome.
   4. Fatigue and pallor.
   5. From examination of the peripheral blood and of a bone marrow aspirate.
   6. 2–3 years
   7. Because immunosuppression renders them liable to potentially fatal infection.
   8. Between 30 and 50 per cent.

2
- correct
- incorrect
- incorrect
- correct
- incorrect

- incorrect
- correct
- incorrect
- correct
- incorrect

H. Understanding discourse

Listen to part of a conversation between a doctor and a patient in a hospital ward.

Dr Jones: Good morning, Mr Smith.

Mr Smith: Good morning, Dr Jones.

Dr Jones: I've come to see you about your operation tomorrow. Do you understand what it will involve?

Mr Smith: I know that you're going to open me up and take a look at my intestines.

Dr Jones: That's right. We're going to put you to sleep with a general anaesthetic and have a look to see what's wrong. But before we can do this, we need to have your consent in writing.

Mr Smith: Oh, yes. What do I have to write?

Dr Jones: You don't have to write anything. You simply sign this standard consent form. Here let me read it to you:
   'I, Fred Smith of 23 Horton Road, Newchurch, hereby consent to undergo the operation of "Laparotomy. ? proceed", the nature and effect of which have been explained to me by Dr Jones. I also consent to such further or alternative operative measures as may be found to be necessary during the course of the operation and to the administration of a general, local or other anaesthetic for any of these purposes. No assurance has been given to me that the operation will be performed by any particular surgeon.'
   There! That's all there is to it. Have you got any questions?

Mr Smith: No, not really. But to tell the truth, I don't really understand all of it. For instance, this part. 'I hereby consent to undergo the operation of "laparotomy. ? proceed". What does that mean?

Dr Jones: That means that we'll take a look inside your abdomen, and examine your large intestine to see what's going on, and what should be done about it.

Mr Smith: And what exactly am I consenting to if I agree to "? proceed"?

Dr Jones: It means that if there is a cancer, we'll remove part of your intestine and do what's best. It might mean that we would have to create a colostomy, in other words create an opening between the intestine and the outside through your abdominal wall.

Mr Smith: You mean that I'll go to sleep not knowing whether I'm going to wake up with half my intestine gone and a colostomy bag stuck to my belly?

Dr Jones: I suppose you could put it like that. But I assure you that it's a perfectly normal way of going about things.

Mr Smith: I'm not sure I like the sound of it. And what about the next sentence? "I also consent to such further or alternative operative measures as may be found to be necessary during the course of the operation." That sounds as if I am agreeing to anything at all being done to me.

Dr Jones: Well, it doesn't really mean that. It's only meant to cover the unexpected, and nothing's done that isn't strictly necessary.

Mr Smith: Then there's the last sentence: "No assurance has been given to me that the operation will be performed by any particular surgeon." Does that mean that it might be performed by the most junior surgeon, who's just been on call for 120 hours?

Dr Jones: Yes, it could mean that. But I think the boss wants to do your operation himself. No guarantees of course.

Mr Smith: I'm not very happy about all this. Have I any choice?

Dr Jones: You've always got a choice. It has to be your decision in the end. But if there's a chance of it being cancer, it's best to get it dealt with as soon as possible.

Mr Smith: Alright then. I'll just have to put myself in your hands. Where do I sign?

KEY

1 – To undergo the operation of "laparotomy. ? proceed"
   – To any other measures found to be necessary
   – To the administration of any type of anaesthetic
   – To accept that there is no assurance that the operation will be performed by any particular surgeon.

2 He will be given a general anaesthetic and his abdomen will be opened. His large intestine will be examined. It may be necessary to remove part of the intestine and to create a colostomy, an opening from the intestine to the outside through the abdominal wall.

3 No exact key is possible. This is a contentious and topical issue. Which should come first, the convenience of the doctor or the convenience of the patient? Do some doctors see a patient simply as a case of a disease, rather than a person? Should patients still be expected to trust their doctor unquestioningly?

4 No key is possible.

UNIT 12: SURGERY

A. Understanding a printed text (1)

KEY

1 A protrusion of a viscus or part of a viscus through its coverings into an abnormal situation.
2 Reducible, irreducible, strangulated.
3 A reducible lump with a cough impulse.
4 A femoral hernia.
5 Excision of the sac and closure of the femoral canal.

B. Check your understanding

KEY

1 Parietal peritoneum.
2 Umbilical.
3 Chronic cough, constipation, urinary obstruction, distension of the abdomen with ascites, gross obesity, muscle wasting in cachexia.
4 Gangrene and perforation.

5 Severe pain in the hernia of sudden onset, central abdominal colicky pain, vomiting, distension and absolute constipation.

6 A plug of fat and a lymph node.

7 Inguinal hernias.

8 The femoral artery.

9 Above and medial to the pubic tubercle.

10 Only a part of the wall of the gut is involved.

C. Increase your vocabulary

KEY

1
- protrude
- constrict
- reduce
- adhere
- distend
- obstruct
- excise
- penetrate
- strangulate

2 1e, 2l, 3k, 4b, 5o, 6m, 7n, 8a, 9j, 10f, 11d, 12c, 13i, 14g, 15h

3 Viscera, diverticula, haematomata.

D. Check your grammar

KEY

1 internal, lateral, superior, distal

2 No key is possible.

E. Understanding a lecture

TAPESCRIPT

You will now hear part of a lecture on the language of surgery.

The subject of today's lecture is 'the language of surgery' and in it we shall look at common descriptive terms used by surgeons. First of all look at the first diagram (a) in your books. This shows how the abdomen is often respresented in medical notes. The six sides represent the borders of the abdomen. The upper two are the costal margins, that is, the lower end of the rib cage. The vertical lines are the lateral edges of the abdomen, and the two lines forming a 'V' shape at the bottom are the inguinal ligaments.

▶▶▶

The diagram shows the abdomen divided into eight areas. The central area is the umbilical region. Lateral to this are the right and left flanks. Above the right flank and below the right costal margin is the right upper quadrant. Note that the left side of the diagram as you look at it on the paper represents the right side of the abdomen. Between the right and left upper quadrants lies the epigastrium. Inferior to or below the right and left flanks lie the right iliac fossa and the left iliac fossa. Between these lies the suprapubic area. All these areas are said to have contents; for example, in the right upper quadrant lie the liver and gall bladder. If a patient had an inflammation of the gall bladder, which is known as cholecystitis, you would expect to get pain in this area. Similarly, pain in the right iliac fossa could be caused by appendicitis, as the appendix is found in this region.

▶▶▶

Now let's look at some of the more common terms you will encounter. Words ending in -ostomy, that's O–S–T–O–M–Y, mean 'opening onto the skin'. For example, a colostomy means that the colon is opened onto the skin. Similarly, a gastrojejunostomy is the result of making a communication between the stomach and a loop of jejunum. Another common ending is -plasty, that's P–L–A–S–T–Y. This means refashioning something to make it work. For example, pyloroplasty means surgically altering the size of the pylorus, which is the outlet of the stomach. The ending -ectomy,

that's E–C–T–O–M–Y, means cutting something out. For instance, appendicectomy literally means cutting out the appendix. The last ending that I'll mention today is -otomy, O–T–O–M–Y, which means cutting something open; laparotomy means cutting open the abdomen. If you remember what these endings mean, you will be able to understand words which contain them, even if the words are totally new to you.

▶▶▶

Now look at the second diagram. This shows a number of lines which represent incisions. An incision is an opening cut in the skin — in this case in the anterior abdominal wall — through which an operation is performed. Particular incisions are used for particular operations. For example, the incision used for extracting the gall bladder (the operation of cholecystectomy) is an oblique incision below the right costal margin. It is called Kocher's incision after the surgeon who first described it. The mid-line or laparotomy incision lies in the midline, as its name suggests, although the cut by-passes the umbilicus. The Pfannenstiel incision is a horizontal line lying across the suprapubic region. The grid-iron used for appendicectomies lies in the right iliac fossa. The right paramedian incision lies to the right of the mid-line. The loin incision is used in renal, or kidney, surgery and lies in the upper quadrant and flank regions. Nearly all abdominal operations will use one of these incisions that I've listed.

KEY

1

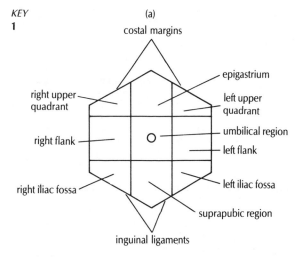

(a)

2
- inflammation of the gall bladder; right upper quadrant
- right iliac fossa

3
- opening onto the skin
- refashioning something to make it work
- cutting something out, e.g. appendicectomy
- cutting something open, e.g. laparotomy.

4

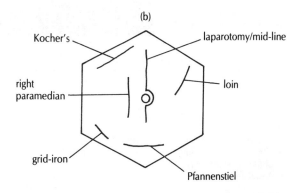

(b)

G. Check your understanding

- incorrect
- incorrect
- correct
- incorrect
- correct

- incorrect
- incorrect
- correct
- incorrect
- incorrect

H. Understanding discourse

TAPESCRIPT
You will now hear a radio reporter interviewing a surgeon who is performing an appendicectomy.

Reporter: Today's edition of 'Your life in their hands' comes to you direct from the operating theatre at St Stephen's Hospital, where we are about to witness the removal of an appendix. The patient is already anaesthetised on the operating table. The surgeon and assisting nurses are coming into the operating theatre, dressed in sterile green gowns with gloves, caps and face masks. I shall now approach the operating table where, under the glare of the lights, the surgeon is preparing to make his first incision. Mr Cutter, perhaps you could guide our listeners.

Mr Cutter: Certainly. As you see, the patient has been covered in sterile drapes, leaving exposed only the lower right quadrant of the abdomen. The skin has been cleaned with iodine, which accounts for the orange colour. I shall now take a scalpel and make a small incision about six centimetres long. This is known as a grid-iron incision and is made at a point two-thirds of the way from the umbilicus to the anterior superior iliac spine. Knife, please, nurse . . . . There, one stroke of the knife takes us through the skin and the yellow fat layer. You can see the white of the muscle sheath glistening below. Diathermy, please, nurse.

Reporter: What's the diathermy, Mr Cutter? Could you explain its function to us?

Mr Cutter: It's a simple idea, really. It's a way of stopping bleeding from small blood vessels by burning with an electric current. I touch the metal probe to the bleeding point and press a pedal with my foot. There. You see? A short frying sound and an acrid smell of scorching flesh, and the bleeding stops.

Reporter: What's the next step?

Mr Cutter: The nurse is stretching the edges of the incision apart with instruments known as retractors. I'm cutting through the muscle layers, stopping the bleeding points as I go. We've now arrived at a thick white sheath of connective tissue, known as fascia. We cut through that, and below is the peritoneum, which is the thin membrane that lines the inside of the abdominal cavity. I'll hold it with my forceps and make a small cut. There we are. We're into the abdominal cavity, and you can see the intestines sliding against one another as the patient's diaphram moves with respiration. I'm now going to reach inside with my fingers and locate the caecum. Yes, I've got it. And behind it should be the appendix. Yes, there we are. I'll pull it out through the incision. Non-crushing clamp, please, nurse.

Reporter: Mr Cutter has now produced through the incision an angry, reddened structure about the size of a little finger. Is that an abnormal appendix, Mr Cutter?

Mr Cutter: Yes, indeed it is. It's markedly inflamed and certainly needs to come out.

Reporter: What's the procedure from now on?

Mr Cutter: I'll tie off the blood vessels on the exterior of the appendix individually with lengths of silk. Then I'll tie the appendix itself off from the bowel and simply chop it off. I'll then invert the stump into the body of the bowel and close it with a purse-string stitch. Then I'll sew up each of the layers that we cut through, finishing with the skin.

Reporter: It seems a very straightforward operation, Mr Cutter. It doesn't take long and, dare I say it, there's not too much blood. Are there ever any complications?

Mr Cutter: It's a simple operation that even the most junior doctor can do under supervision. But, of course, difficulties can arise. Sometimes the appendix is difficult to find, and sometimes it's stuck down with inflammation. And this patient's quite thin. In a fat person, it's much more complicated, because you have to operate through a long tunnel of fat.

Reporter: Thank you, Mr Cutter. And now, as the surgeon closes his incision, that's the end of this week's programme and I'm returning you to the studio.

1 Surgeon and nurses wear sterile gowns, gloves, caps and masks; patient is covered with sterile drapes; skin is cleaned with iodine.
2 Skin; fat; muscle; fascia; peritoneum.
3 Electrocautery — a method of stopping bleeding of small blood vessels by burning with an electric current. The bleeding point is touched with a metal probe and the current is operated with a foot pedal.
4 Lots of blood.
5 The appendix may be difficult to find; it may be stuck down with inflammation; the patient may be fat.

UNIT 13: ANATOMY

A. Understanding a printed text (1)

1 2.5 cm.
2 Sclera and cornea, the uveal tract, the retina.
3 Astigmatism.
4 Nil. The cornea has no blood supply.
5 The ciliary and conjunctival branches of the opthalmic division of the trigeminal nerve.
6 A ball and socket joint.

B. Check your understanding

1 The superior and inferior orbital margins.
2 The lens.
3 The lamina cribrosa.
4 Glaucoma; raised intra-ocular pressure.
5 The cornea.
6 The cornea and the lens.
7 Leprosy and syphilis.

8 Because the absence of a blood supply to the cornea prevents the lymphocytes reaching the tissue.

9 Injury by foreign particles leading to corneal ulceration.

10 The centre.

C. Increase your vocabulary

KEY

1 a. junction, branches
  b. sphere, globe, curvature
  c. capsule, sheath
  d. plane, vertical, horizontal
  e. margin, border

2 ● extends
  ● receives
  ● lies
  ● is covered
  ● is separated
  ● enters
  ● is divided
  ● is filled
  ● projects

D. Check your grammar

KEY

1 of; in; of; in; by; of; by; from; by; around; to
2 through; by; in; from; along/through; to

E. Understanding a lecture

TAPESCRIPT

Listen to the lecture on the anatomy of the kidney.

Today, I'm going to talk about the anatomy of the kidneys. First of all, where are they? Well, the kidneys are paired structures: that means there are two of them. They lie on the posterior abdominal wall, one on each side of the vertebral column. And they're retroperitoneal, in other words they're situated behind the peritoneum, which lines the abdominal cavity. They're about three and a half vertebrae long, and the left kidney is slightly higher than the right kidney. That's because the right kidney is pushed down by the liver. In fact, neither kidney is completely still. They move up and down with respiration, by about the length of one vertebra.

▶▶▶

What about the size and shape of the kidneys? Well, the kidneys are bean-shaped, with the indented part, which is known as the hilum, turned towards the mid-line of the body. Each kidney measures about 12 centimetres by 7 centimetres by 3 centimetres, but of course there's quite a lot of variation from person to person. In the male, they weight about 160 grammes each, but in the female they're slightly lighter. Both kidneys are embedded in fat and covered in a layer of fascia which holds them in place.

▶▶▶

Next, we'll look at the structures which enter or leave the kidney at the hilum. First of all there is the ureter. This is the tube that takes the urine produced by the kidney down to the bladder. Then there are the renal artery and the renal vein. The renal artery is quite a large artery and comes directly off the aorta. The veins are similarly large and drain into the large vein known as the superior vena cava. Although these connections are large, they're not very complicated. So the plumbing involved in removing a kidney and replacing it with another is reasonably simple. The problem with kidney transplants is the phenomenon known as rejection. The body will turn against the transplanted kidney unless it is closely matched to the tissue type of the recipient.

▶▶▶

Finally, what's actually inside the kidney? What does it consist of? In gross terms, if you slice a kidney lengthwise, there are two main layers visible. The outer layer is known as the cortex and the layer inside the cortex is called the medulla. At a microscopic level, each kidney contains about a million of a structure known as a nephron. This is a long thin tube into which liquid is filtered out of the blood. Some of this liquid is reabsorbed again from the tube. The rest flows down eventually to reach the ureter, and forms the urine. The actual structure of the nephron is quite complicated and will have to wait for another lecture.

KEY

1 *Section 1*
  ● because the right kidney is pushed down by the liver
  ● respiration
  Section 2
  ● 12 × 7 × 3 cm
  ● about 160 grammes
  Section 3
  ● the ureter, the renal artery and the renal vein
  ● the superior vena cava
  Section 4
  ● the cortex and the medulla
  ● about one million

2 No key is possible.

G. Check your understanding

KEY

1 The hip and buttock.
2 Ilium, ischium, pubis.
3 The perineum.
4 The tibia and the patella.
5 The greater trochanter of the femur.
6 The tibia and the fibula.
7 Tibia, fibula and talus.
8 The navicular bone.
9 One.
10 The patella.

H. Understanding discourse

TAPESCRIPT

Listen to a conversation between a new student and an older colleague about ways of learning anatomy.

Younger student: What I don't understand is how anyone can possibly be expected to learn so much information. It's just lists of facts completely devoid of ideas. It's mindless. It's completely impossible.

Older student: I felt like that too during my first term of anatomy. In a way, you're absolutely right. It can be completely mindless and quite impossible.

Younger student: But then how do people ever get through it all? How did you manage when you did it?

Older student: One has to adopt certain learning strategies in order to get by. Haven't you ever wondered how memory experts in the music hall used to make their living?

Younger student: No, I can't say I have. I suppose they were all either terribly clever or totally dishonest.

Older student: I don't think that's true at all. They simply used memory techniques, such as mnemonics.

Younger student: Mn . . . what?

Older student:	Mnemonics. M–N–E–M–O–N–I–C–S.
Younger student:	And what are they?
Older student:	I'll give you an example. If you want to remember the five terminal branches of the facial nerve, you have to be able to think them up correctly and in the right order: temporal, zygomatic, buccal, mandibular, cervical.
Younger student:	That's just the sort of thing I can't do.
Older student:	Well, I can remember them easily, 'cause instead of trying to remember the list, I just remember the sentence 'two zebras bit my cat'. Then I take the first letter of each word and work it out from there. It's a much easier way of doing it.
Younger student:	Sounds pretty weird to me.
Older student:	But it works.
Younger student:	What other tricks have you got up your sleeve? Or is that where you hide the answers when you go into exams?
Older student:	Well, another important thing in anatomy is to use lots of pictures. It's much easier to take things in if you can see them. Pictures are easier to remember than lists of words. Then there are things called sieves.

Younger student:	What are they?
Older student:	Well, you split everything up into flow diagrams. It's really a form of classification. If you impose a logical structure on the information, it makes it easier to learn. Also, it's an awful lot quicker to revise from a flow diagram than it is if you're just faced with a solid chunk of prose.
Younger student:	So that's all there is to it, then? Is that the secret?
Older student:	That was just a few things to help you along. But it's no substitute for hard work. The only way to keep on remembering things is to revise them frequently.
Younger student:	Thanks. I'm not sure whether to feel encouraged or discouraged. I'll go away and give it a try.

KEY

1 He is having difficulty in learning so much information.
2 Mnemonics; illustrations; sieves (flow diagrams).
3 The terminal branches of the facial nerve.
4 Imposing a logical order on information makes it easier to remember; it is easier to revise from flow diagrams than from paragraphs of prose.
5 Frequent revision.

UNIT 14: MEDICAL RESEARCH

A. Understanding a printed text (1)

KEY

1 A letter.
2 The psychiatric wing of a London teaching hospital.
3 A histogram.
4 Fifteen months.
5 There is a significant positive correlation between the number of violent incidents and the proportion of agency staff.

B. Check your understanding

KEY

1 Because of an increase in violent incidents on the acute admission ward.
2 Characteristics of the ward population and of the staff that might be associated with the increase in violence.
3 At night.
4 Kendall's rank correlation.
5 It remained steady.
6 It halved.
7 Schizophrenia.
8 No.
9 $p < 0.001$.

C. Increase your vocabulary

KEY

1 ● halved
  ● doubled
  ● trebled
  ● hazard
  ● shift
2 1e, 2c, 3f, 4a, 5b, 6d.
3 No key is possible.

D. Check your grammar

KEY

1 ● If more money were made available for health services, the health of the population would improve.
  ● If people smoked less, mortality from respiratory and cardiovascular disease would decline.
  ● If we eliminated poverty, fewer doctors would be needed.
  ● If kidney dialysis was cheaper, more people would be treated.
  ● If the theory was true, we would soon be rich.
2 A choice of expression is possible for each answer, as given in the examples in the Students' Book.
3 The sentences should be completed as in the example:
  ● less than 1 in 100
  ● less than 1 in 10
  ● less than 1 in 100,000.

E. Understanding a lecture

TAPESCRIPT

Good morning, ladies and gentlemen. Today, I'm going to talk about how to do research in medicine. We'll take the subject step by step and I'll explain how to set up a research project. Right, then. The first thing you have to do is find a subject that interests you and think of an idea. This usually involves thinking of some problem that you would like to look at or test in some way. You may find your ideas from what is going on around you, or you may develop them from reading textbooks or other people's research. Secondly, you have to formulate a testable hypothesis! This means that you make a specific statement about the subject that you are going to try and prove or disprove in your research. At this point, it's important to find out exactly what is already known about the subject. So the third thing you have to do is a literature search. You can begin by looking in textbooks. Then you can ask the advice of someone who specialises in the subject. You can look in all the specialist journals to see what others have written, and these days there are special computer programmes to help you find what you're looking for. The literature search is important because there's no point in doing something that has been done fifty times before. It's difficult to think of completely new ideas and often you may find that someone else has thought of them first.

▶▶▶

Let's assume that you've got a testable hypothesis and that it hasn't been looked at before. Now you have to design a way of testing it. You have to decide exactly what you are going to measure and what method you are going to use to measure it. You've also got to think about how many subjects you will need and how long you're going to do it for. There is no point in planning a huge project, because it's unlikely that you'll ever have the time or the money to finish it. Looking at the literature will help you design a method. When you've got this far, you should write a protocol. This is a detailed written plan of your research. You can use it for the next two steps in setting up your project: these are applying for ethical approval and finding funding. If the project involves forms of treatment, such as drugs, it is usually necessary to seek the approval of a special body which looks at the ethics of the experiment and protects the interests of the patients. As far as funding is concerned, most research costs money. You may have to pay people to carry out the research, to take part in it, or to analyse the results. Even simple things like paper and getting things typed cost money.

▶▶▶

At this point, you should run a pilot project. This means that you do a limited smaller version of your project in order to see what difficulties you are going to have. Often these are things that you hadn't thought of. The pilot study can be very useful in allowing you to make changes to your method before it is too late. Finally, you get to run the main project and the hard work really begins. But what about when you've managed to gather all your data? Well, you still have to analyse them and work out what they mean. Then you have to try and write them up in a publishable form. This may take as long as all the other steps put together. And there's no guarantee that all your hard work is going to produce anything interesting. It can be a hard life doing research.

KEY

1 How to do research in medicine.
2 Think of an idea; form a testable hypothesis; conduct a literature search; design a way of testing your hypothesis; write a protocol; apply for ethical approval; find funding; run a pilot project; run the main project; analyse the data; write them up in a publishable form.
3 To make sure that your idea hasn't already been thought of by someone else; to help design the experimental method.
4 Because you won't have the time or the money to finish it.
5 To discover hidden difficulties before it is too late to correct them.
6 If the student is unable to think of an idea, a simple one should be provided by the teacher. The student should describe how he will go about things following as far as possible the pattern set out in the answer to (2) above.

G. Check your understanding

KEY

1
- incorrect
- correct
- correct
- incorrect
- correct

- incorrect
- correct
- correct
- correct
- correct

2
- The Birmingham births register of the university department of social medicine.

- Because these data were incomplete at the time of the study.
- Because data on ethnic origin are not routinely collected when births are registered in Britain.
- A different socio-economic distribution from that among other ethnic groups and a lower mean birth weight.
- It might provide aetiological clues.

H. Understanding discourse

TAPESCRIPT
You will now hear a telephone conversation between two hospital doctors.

(Ring ring)
Bob: Five-one-two-three-seven.
Alec: Hello, Bob? It's Alec.
Bob: Hello, Alec. How are you?
Alec: Fine, thanks. Listen, I was wondering if you could give me some advice.
Bob: Certainly, if I can. What's the problem?
Alec: Well, I hear you're chairman of the ethical committee these days, and I thought I'd sound you out about a project we're just setting up.
Bob: Yes. Why not? What is it?
Alec: It's a trial of a new antidepressant drug. The company that makes it have offered the department a lot of money to test it out against a standard preparation.
Bob: I see. Sounds simple enough. Where's the difficulty?
Alec: Well, they want a three-way double-blind trial with the third group being put on placebo.
Bob: You mean that a third of the patients won't be receiving an active preparation and you won't know which third?
Alec: That's right. And we want to use a group of patients with severe depression.
Bob: Well, you'll have to make sure that they're properly supervised. You don't want any suicides in your placebo group. I don't think you'd better include out-patients in the trial. Otherwise, I doubt there'll be many problems in getting it through the committee.
Alec: The thing is that we would want to use it on patients who are sectioned.
Bob: You mean you'd want to try it out on patients who are held against their will in the psychiatric unit?
Alec: Yeah, that's it.
Bob: Well. I'm not sure about that in the current climate. It wouldn't have been a problem a few years ago, but these days everyone's really concerned about the question of consent.
Alec: Yes, I realise that. But we were hoping to get round it by only using sectioned patients who give their consent to take part in the trial.
Bob: Wait a minute. That sounds a little too clever. If you're keeping them in hospital against their will, it's because you believe they're not fit to judge whether they should be in hospital or not so how then can you say that they're fit to consent to take part in a drug trial?
Alec: Well, you know. Patients never really understand what their treatment involves anyway.
Bob: I know that and you know that. But it's just not good enough these days. I'm afraid you may have to drop the idea of using sectioned patients. You can put in an application to the committee if you like, but I think it would probably be rejected.
Alec: OK. Thanks for the advice: That's very helpful. I'll take it back to the drug company and they'll just have to revise their ideas.
Bob: Any time, Alec. By the way, will you be coming to the inaugural lecture next week?

Alec: Yes, I'll probably see you there.
Bob: Cheerio, then.
Alec: Cheerio.

KEY

1 1. Psychiatric patients.
2. Chairman of the ethical committee.
3. A trial of a new antidepressant against a standard preparation and placebo, on a double-blind basis.
4. Severely depressed patients may end up being treated with

placebo; Alec wants to use patients detained in hospital against their will.
5. Bob advises Alec to abandon the idea of using detained patients.

2 This exercise can be written or form the basis for a class discussion. Examples of the benefits of such trials are the fact that effective drugs cannot be developed in any other way, and the financial benefit accruing to underfinanced hospital departments. Objections are likely to include the idea of ill people being used as guinea pigs and being treated with preparations that may not work, or even with inactive placebos.

UNIT 15: THE FUTURE OF MEDICINE

A. Understanding a printed text (1)

KEY

1 Cholera, smallpox, puerperal fever, surgical infections, pneumonia, tuberculosis and typhoid.
2 Sulphonamides.
3 It has ensured that dying costs vastly more than it did 25 years ago.
4 An applied science.
5 'Can we demonstrate that this new thing is better for the patient in terms of cure, relief or comfort?'

B. Check your understanding

KEY

1 1. Because of major advances in the prevention and treatment of infectious diseases.
2. 2.7 years.
3. Peptic ulcer and renal failure.
4. H_2 antagonists; renal dialysis and transplantation.
5. About 3%. 8.75% in the USA, 5.75% in Britain.
6. To improve the lot of human beings unfortunate enough to suffer disease.
7. Scholars should only study problems of which the solution will help mankind.
2 No key is possible.

C. Increase your vocabulary

KEY

1 ● ingenious
● pious
● materialise
● anticipated
2 1d, 2a, 3b, 4c, 5e.
3 ● combat, conquer, rout
● pour, flood

D. Check your grammar

KEY

The words/phrases can be omitted in 2, 4, 5, 6.

E. Understanding a lecture

TAPESCRIPT

Good afternoon! Today, I'm going to talk about some problems affecting health care systems in Western countries. Whilst I'll concentrate on issues affecting the British health service, other countries are confronting the same difficulties to a greater or lesser degree.

▶▶▶

First amongst these are the demographic changes occurring in the West. As the average life expectancy slowly increases and the birth rate stabilises at a low level, the result is a shift in the age profile of the population. In other words, more people are old these days. The elderly, who no longer contribute to the creation of wealth, form a greater proportion of the population. They are intensive users of health care resources. The proportion of young people, whose tax payments finance all forms of welfare provision, is at the same time decreasing. The danger is that there may not be enough money available to support health care systems in their current form. This has resulted in a fundamental reconsideration of systems of health provision.

▶▶▶

In Britain, recent government dogma has been that people should be encouraged to pay for their health care, rather than expect it from the state system. Some people could certainly afford to pay for health care, but the people who need the care most, such as the old and the chronically ill, are the ones least able to buy the care they need. And there are two, more fundamental, reasons why an increase in the private sector cannot provide a realistic solution to the funding problem. The first is that increasing needs have to be met with increased resources. A switch from public to private finance would not increase the overall total spent on care. And this is less in Britain as a percentage of gross national product than in most other West European countries or in the USA. The second reason is one of efficiency. It is a simple fact that the public health care system in Britain is more efficient and cost-effective than any other health system, public or private. And it's noticeable that private health care companies are not interested in competing over most of the field of health care, because there is no money in it.

▶▶▶

There is, however, another more forward-looking approach to health care. This is the idea of prevention. If sickness and disease are expensive, then it will be cheaper to prevent them where this can be done. The initiation of preventative policies requires major changes in society with attention turned to such matters as nutrition, housing, environment and working conditions. Unfortunately, this conflicts with the interests of businessmen and politicians who deal principally with short-term profit rather than long-term gain. At present, the political will to bring about social change in the interests of health is largely lacking. But the realities of the situation suggest that it is unlikely to remain so.

KEY

1 Some problems affecting health care systems in Western countries.
2 Demographic changes; public or private finance; prevention.
3 The proportion of elderly in the population is increasing, whereas the proportion of young is decreasing.
4 There are fewer young to provide for the increasing needs of the old.
5 The people who need the care most are the ones who could not afford to pay for it; increasing needs must be met by increasing resources, not a change in source of existing levels of funding; the public health care system in Britain is more efficient and cost-effective than any other system; private health care companies aren't interested in large areas of health care, because there is no money in them.
6 Nutrition, housing, the environment, working conditions.

G. Check your understanding

KEY

1 ● Bankruptcy.
  ● The amount of money and energy spent on terminal care.
  ● Using expensive technology which is of little effect, to collude with the refusal of patients to accept that they must in the end die.
  ● Thirty thousand dollars.
  ● That provided by a district hospital.
2 No key is possible. The author clearly favours the white (or red) arrow. Few coherent counter-arguments are possible; they concern the natural tendency of the strong to survive at the expense of the weak, or the individual's right to choose.

H. Understanding discourse

TAPESCRIPT
You will now hear part of a discussion amongst the members of a health district committee called to discuss a financial crisis.

Chairman: Quiet, please! I'd like to call this meeting to order. We've got a lot to get through and the sooner we get started, the better. I'll presume there are no corrections to the Minutes of the previous meeting unless someone interrupts me now. Any matters arising? No? Then, let's get straight on with item one on the agenda, the financial shortfall. Over to you, Mr Treasurer.
Treasurer: Thank you, Mr Chairman. I'm sure you've all read my report which was circulated with the agenda for this meeting. In short, the health district is faced with an overspend of twenty million pounds in the current financial year. There's no chance of any more money coming from government. So, unless we make sharp

cuts in next year's budget, the hospital will go bankrupt. Now I've set up a number of proposals for areas in which to make financial readjustments.
Member 1: . . . otherwise known as cuts.
Treasurer: If I may continue! Let's start with the first one: the proposed closure of a further two surgical wards and the rescheduling of the new cardiac unit.
Member 1: I'd like to make a point here, Mr Chairman. We've already had two surgical wards closed for six months. Why close another two? The surgical unit has never been more efficient. We've responded to your previous calls, and we've treated twice as many patients as last year with half as many beds.
Treasurer: Well, that's the problem. You've been too efficient and treated so many people that your costs have actually increased. Unless you become less efficient, we'll simply have to close more beds.
Member 1: But we've dramatically improved our service to patients. Isn't that what we were asked to do? Don't the patients come first?
Treasurer: In general, yes. But in this instance, the budget comes first. If the hospital goes bankrupt, we won't be able to provide any service to patients at all.
Member 1: And what's the point in spending all that capital on the new cardiac unit if we can't afford to open it?
Treasurer: Capital expenditure comes out of a different budget from running costs, and it's not what's on the agenda for today. Let's get on to the second item: a proposed halving of the budget for community services.
Member 2: Well, here I really must protest, Mr Chairman. We're supposed to be entering the age of community care. All our long-stay hospitals are closing and the occupants are being transferred back to the community. How are they going to be cared for if there are no services available?
Treasurer: Well, the community care policy is not one that we invented. The families will just have to do more, and the rest of the burden will fall on social services rather than on the hospital budget. The sad fact is that we've got to make cuts somewhere.
Member 3: You mean that community care mainly involves the old and the mentally ill, and they don't carry much political weight.
Treasurer: I mean that desirable as such services may be, they don't directly save lives, unlike most of our other specialities.
Member 2: But all that will happen is that the situation will break down at home and the patients will end up coming into our hospital as emergencies.
Treasurer: Perhaps. Perhaps not. Since we have so many beds closed, such patients would have to go to other hospitals anyway, so it won't be out of our budget! Or it may not happen until the financial year after next, when we may have more resources to deal with it.
Member 2: That's hardly the caring voice of the medical profession.
Treasurer: I sympathise with your comments. But that's all politics. My role is simply one of management. Given current financial circumstances, we have no choice, I'm afraid, I don't like it any more than you do, but that's the way it is. Or can any of you offer an alternative solution? . . . (silence) . . . Then, I take it that the decision is made. Thank you, Mr Chairman.

KEY
1 1. The financial shortfall.
  2. The district is faced with an overspend of twenty million pounds.
  3. Surgical beds; community care.

4. The surgical unit has dramatically increased its efficiency and managed to treat twice as many patients with half as many beds. As a result the cost of running the unit has gone up, although the cost of treating each patient has gone down.
5. Patients in the community who would have been supported by the cut services will present to the hospital as emergencies. The Treasurer suggests that they may have to go to other hospitals, because there will not be enough beds in this one. The problem may not occur until the financial year after next.

2 The discusson caricatured in this discourse is a very real and common one in health districts throughout Britain. The points of view put forward represent in many ways the state of a wider debate. Whilst neither side is necessarily wrong, it can be remarked that the Treasurer is perhaps using the financial absolutes as a defence against confronting the real meaning of the cuts. And the dissenting members are simply objecting to change, instead of accepting its inevitability and seeking to seize the initiative in determining its direction.